There Are Survivors:

The Michael Cuccione Story

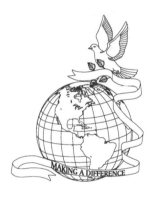

Jane MacSporran & Michael Cuccione

Canadian Cataloguing in Publication Data
Cuccione, Michael, 1985–
There are survivors
ISBN 0-9683188-0-0
1. Cuccione, Michael, 1985– 2. Cancer--Patients--Biography
I. MacSporran, Jane, 1930– II.Title.
RC265.6.C82A3 1998   362.1'96994'0092   C98-910085-5

Production Manager: Diana C. Douglas
Editors: Charlene L. Dryburgh, Julia M. Schoennagel
Text Design: Fiona Raven
Cover Design: Andrew Johnstone
Cover Photograph: Tonino Guzzo
First printing March 1998
10 9 8 7 6 5 4 3 2 1

The information within this book is based on personal experience,
and may not necessarily reflect that of other individuals. Consult
your physician before employing any of the products or treatments
described herein. This book is sold on the understanding that the
publisher, editors, producer, and distributors are not engaged in
rendering medical or professional service.

The authors gratefully acknowledge the permission
received to reprint the lyrics and photographs
included in this book.

MAKING A DIFFERENCE PUBLISHING
P.O. Box 31081, 8 - 2929 St. Johns Street
Port Moody, BC Canada V3H 4T4
Fax (604) 552-2808

Printed in Canada

"Michael is irresistible. A kid who overcame disease and rose to prominence overnight as a child speaker, singer, writer and celebrity. His story WOWs my soul. I've watched him captivate audiences of thousands with as much charisma and style as Frank Sinatra.

His story will touch your heart, soul and improve your experience. This book will positively impact you and your future. Michael's story is unforgettable."

Mark Victor Hansen, Co-author
New York Times #1 Best-selling *Chicken Soup for the Soul* series

"Michael Cuccione is an inspirational and exceptional child. God chooses people and sometimes chooses children to teach people and other children about Love, Light, Leadership, and Priorities. Michael has definitely been chosen by God to help us all. God has blessed Michael and I am proud to have him as a friend. Keep smiling, Michael."

David Hasselhoff, Producer/Actor/Singer
Baywatch series

Dedication

This book is dedicated to Melinda Rose Hathaway
(May 19, 1981–September 15, 1996) and to the special people,
including all the patients of British Columbia's Children's
Hospital, who came into my life during my illness.

I met Melinda while both of us were receiving cancer
treatments in B.C.'s Children's Hospital. We felt an immediate
connection which continues even now through our websites.

Melinda's home page is on the Internet at **http://
www.monkeyboy.com/Melinda/**. Her stated purpose for
creating her home page was: *"To help provide other Cancer
Kids and their caregivers with hope, with important information
that they might be looking for, and with contact to other Cancer
Kids, caregivers, and cancer related sites all over the world."* She
did this when she knew that her time on earth was very short.

I created my website to inform people about important
events that are taking place in my life: the research that is
being carried on through the money raised by the Michael
Cuccione Foundation; the benefit of herbs in helping to
maintain my bodily health; and the latest developments in
cancer treatments that are being revealed through the media.

My website can be found at **www.makingadifference.org**
or e-mail me at either **love@makingadifference.org** or at
support@makingadifference.org. I will endeavour to reply
to all my e-mail.

Michael Cuccione

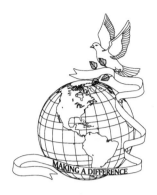

Preface

Michael Cuccione has survived two bouts with cancer and the treatments that go with this diagnosis. He has become a young man with a mission to help raise the funds necessary to find a cure for cancer.

This book was written from the combined journals of Michael and me. I am Michael's Grandmother, Jane MacSporran. I began to keep a journal when Michael was first diagnosed with cancer. Initially, it was a form of therapy, helping me deal with the intensity of the situation. I had no thought of it being published as a book. Then, Michael made his commitment to help stop the pain and suffering of others. He wrote songs, both while he was in the hospital and recovering, and ultimately produced a CD called *Make a Difference*. As he began to travel to promote his cause, speaking to large audiences and being on radio and TV, he began keeping a journal of his own experiences. The journal also helped him to meet one of his school requirements. Eventually, we decided to integrate our journals and write this story. We also reviewed videos of Michael's public appearances, and interviewed each other and family members. The result is this book.

Michael and I chose the title, *There Are Survivors: The Michael Cuccione Story*. We feel that whether or not people survive serious illnesses, they are survivors. Those who live have managed to overcome their illnesses. Those who die still survive in the memories of those who love them.

They survive through what they accomplished while alive and through the people who carry on their work. Family and friends who must cope with the suffering are also survivors.

Our intention in publishing Michael's story is to continue to raise awareness of the need to find a cure for cancer. Michael's goal is to bring people together in this cause. As he says, "One person can only do so much, but together we can make a difference."

I am glad that I kept my journal, for I consider Michael an inspiration to anyone facing adversity. He faced his situation bravely, he kept on being productive, and, to borrow from his song, *Never Give Up*, he never gave up on hope, he never gave up on faith, and he never gave up on love.

Jane MacSporran

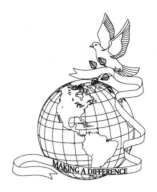

Acknowledgements

I thank God first, for answering my prayers and for giving me the strength to make a difference.

A very special thanks to my mom and dad. You have always been there for me through the good times and the bad times and have supported me in everything I do. I will always love you.

I thank my sister, Sophia, and my brother, Steven, for always praying for me. I know it wasn't easy, but we made it together.

There are not enough words to thank you, Gramma Jane, for your hard work and true dedication to our book. This book will always be very special to me, because someone I love and who felt my pain helped me tell my story.

To my Nonna Anna, Nonno Armando and Great Nonna Rosa: I know you all shed a lot of tears for me and prayed endlessly that I would get through my adversity, and it helped me so much. Thank you, Nonna Anna, for the great food you sent me while I was in the hospital.

I thank all my aunts, uncles and cousins for your love and support for me and my family. It was great to know that we were not alone.

A special thanks to my uncle, Mike Cuccione, Sr. You have always believed in me and are a fantastic role model in my life. You have been incredibly supportive of my cause by helping take my CD across Canada with Burger King.

My never-ending gratitude to Dr. Anderson. You helped to save my life. You went beyond the call of duty by becoming part of our family. We value your on-going support and true friendship.

Thank you to all doctors, nurses and staff at B.C.'s Children's Hospital for your great care.

There are so many more people who have helped me in the past three years, to whom I am very grateful:

My special friends who are no longer with me. God bless them.

Anna Terrana, former MP for East Vancouver, for caring about me and supporting my mission. By organizing the meeting with the Prime Minister of Canada, you helped me to spread my message across the country.

Enrich International for providing me with the products which helped me to recover and maintain my health.

My main sponsors, Burger King Canada, Shoppers Drug Mart, and Save-On Foods. You helped tremendously to further my dream of making a difference by marketing my CDs.

Dana Cole, my voice coach and special friend. I have learned so much from you.

Terry Robotham, whose expertise contributed greatly to the producing, arranging, programming, and engineering of my CD.

Tonino Guzzo, for the fabulous photography on the *Make a Difference* CD and also on the cover of this book. You are always there for me.

Fran Will, R.N., who provided the photographs of Michael she took for a poster presentation of bone marrow transplants.

The board members of the Michael Cuccione Foundation, whose support has been invaluable: Mike Cuccione, Sr., president; Mike Lacombe, vice-president; Maria Marano, secretary; Shelley Young, Patricia Campelletti, Maria Bruneau, Charlene Dryburgh, Domenic and Gloria Cuccione, Chuck Gould, directors; Steven Cuccione, Sr., and Rob Richici, directors-at-large.

The Peoples Network (TPN), who supported me by purchasing my CDs and gave me the pleasure of speaking to thousands of people at their incredible Master Mind convention.

Mark Victor Hansen, co-author of the *Chicken Soup For The Soul* series, books which are filled with inspirational stories. I am very grateful to receive such a powerful endorsement from someone who is so inspirational himself.

David Hasselhoff, Greg Bonann, and the *Baywatch* family. You all made the time I spent at *Baywatch* something I will never forget. David, you believed in me and gave me the opportunity of a lifetime. Thank you for helping me to create a worldwide awareness of my cause. Thank you for your heartfelt words.

Susan Addington, Charlie's mother, who helped me get to know Charlie so that I was able to play his character. Thanks to Charlie, who will never be forgotten. It was an honour to portray Charlie in the *Baywatch* episode.

Rosalie, Dougie, Darlene, and Cliff Gosling, for their friendship and incredible success in fundraising for the Michael Cuccione Foundation.

My many friends in the Italian community, who have surrounded me with love and support from the beginning.

Thank you to Marquis of London for donating the jacket shown in the cover photograph on this book.

Both my grandmother and I thank Diana Douglas and her production team at Peanut Butter Publishing for all their creative time and effort.

Additional thanks to Charlene Dryburgh and Julia Schoennagel for their considerable editing expertise.

I can't begin to express the gratitude I feel for all my supporters who believe in me and my cause, and who have helped me so much with my mission. These people have purchased my CDs, made donations, and organized fundraisers for the Michael Cuccione Foundation.

Michael Cuccione

Contents

Foreword

Michael Cuccione was diagnosed not once, but twice, with cancer. His second diagnosis was of relapsed disease, throwing him into a pitched battle for his life.

Receiving the news that their child has been diagnosed with cancer is the worst possible thing that could happen to a family. They are plunged into a despair from which there seems to be no escape. This was certainly the case for Michael and his family. Michael, however, has fought the odds and successfully undergone surgery, chemotherapy, radiation therapy, and bone marrow transplantation. Through the worst of these times he never complained or showed self-pity. Two things instead were on his mind: that he was going to get better, and that he would make a difference in the lives of others stricken with cancer.

Tremendous strides are being made in the field of childhood cancer treatment and today most children are cured. This was not the case several decades ago, however. Only a small percentage of children were curable and it was generally thought that this situation could not be changed. Through the dedication of scores of physicians, research scientists, and all those involved in the care of childhood cancer, children like Michael can now have hope. However, there are no guarantees for any child or family and much work remains to be done. This work must continue.

Michael is a remarkable young man, and is now the inspiration of many. He and the Michael Cuccione Foundation are making a great contribution to the field of childhood cancer research. Michael deserves full support from all who read this book as he selflessly and tirelessly works to bring his message of hope. He is showing how one individual who cares can truly make a difference.

Ronald Anderson, MD, FRCPC
Associate Professor of Oncology and Pediatrics
Faculty of Medicine, University of Calgary, Alberta

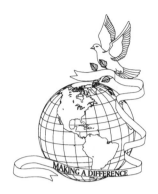

Introduction

Michael Cuccione was born on January 5, 1985, in Burnaby, British Columbia, Canada. He was the middle child born to Domenic and Gloria Cuccione. His older sister, Sophia, was three years old when he was born. His younger brother, Steven, was born three years later. I am the children's grandmother. I moved in with the family when Michael was born and have been with them ever since. Domenic added an in-law suite for me in every new home he built for his family.

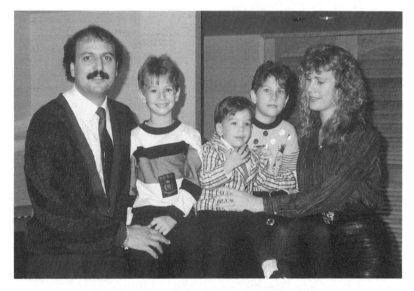

L to R: Domenic, Michael (6 yrs), Steven (2 $\frac{1}{2}$ yrs), Sophia (9 yrs), Gloria.

Michael was greeted by the big loving family of his father, Domenic. We were thrilled to welcome the first boy born into our small but mighty family. Gloria turned to the Roman Catholic faith before she married Domenic, the children are being raised as Roman Catholics. Faith is very important to the family and has been a source of strength to all the family members.

People often ask, "What was Michael like before he developed cancer?" Actually, Michael's personality has changed very little. Just as he is today, Michael was a lively, sociable, talented child, with a great sense of humour and a zest for life. He has always possessed wisdom far beyond his years. He became a high achiever when he started school. A couple of his teachers thought that he talked too much in class; other teachers used this trait to make Michael a class leader. He got along well with other children, but was quite capable of defending himself if he felt that he was being unfairly treated. His outstanding characteristics were, and are, honesty, sincerity, and compassion for others. He is a warm, caring human being.

Life was almost perfect for the Cuccione family. They owned a beautiful home in a good location. His father had a good job in property management. His mother ran her own fashion-wear business several evenings a week so she could be home for the children during the day. The children attended a local school, and were leading happy lives. Michael was receiving call-backs for commercials and was being seriously considered for a TV-series pilot. Sophia, Michael, and Steven were all actively participating in sports. There were many happy get-togethers with the extended family. Love for one another abounded. Life was great.

Then, on July 25, 1994, we received dreadful news. Michael was diagnosed with cancer. He was only nine years old. The next two years were spent trying to save his life.

While Michael was a patient in B.C.'s Children's Hospital, he heard the cries of young children who, like himself, were suffering from cancer. He became determined to do something to put an end to their suffering. He wanted to try to help find a cure for cancer, and this became his mission.

The personal goals he set and has achieved, and how he continues to make a difference, are told in this remarkable story.

Chapter 1

It Can't Be

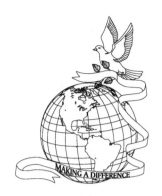

 July 25, 1994

I was feeling very proud of myself. After visiting my son and his wife on Vancouver Island, I had made it home in time for my grandson Steven's sixth birthday. The phone was ringing as I came through the door of my basement apartment in the home of my daughter and son-in-law. I raced to answer it. My daughter Gloria's tearful voice was at the other end of the line. Why was she so upset? Maybe Steven had fallen off his bicycle again?

"What is the matter?" I inquired breathlessly.

"I'm at Children's Hospital in Vancouver."

"Is something wrong with Steven?" I wondered why he would be in Children's Hospital. He must have really injured himself this time!

"It's not Steven, it's Michael."

"Has his strep throat flared up again?"

"No, we are in the oncology clinic," my daughter sobbed.

"What do you mean? What is the oncology clinic?"

"It is the clinic for cancer patients; you should see the poor children in here! They think that Michael has cancer, too!"

"How can that be? He was fine when I saw him a week ago."

"They found two lumps, one on each side of his collar bone. The one on the right is the size of a golf ball and the one on the left is a bit smaller. They think he might have Hodgkin's disease."

"What on earth is Hodgkin's disease?"

"It's a malignant lymph gland disease," responded Gloria.

"Michael can't have cancer. It must be a viral infection or mononucleosis."

"He is with the specialists right now. We will find out at four o'clock whether they think it is Hodgkin's or not. It might even be leukemia."

I ended the telephone call. "I'm coming to the hospital right away. I'll see you in about an hour."

As I drove along, I tried to make sense out of what had happened. Michael could not have cancer! There was no history of cancer in any of our families.

Images of my precious grandson kept flashing before my eyes—his wavy light brown hair, his penetrating green eyes, his ready smile, his loving nature. He and his elder sister, Sophia, bore a strong resemblance to their fair-haired, fair-skinned mother, while Steven had inherited his dark skin and eyes from their Italian father.

Michael seemed to have it all. His scholastic achievement was above average. He had won trophies for his dancing, had his blue belt in karate, and was a born performer, frequently being asked to sing at public functions.

Just that week, he had completed two modelling assignments and had a call-back for a commercial. In addition, a director had arranged for him to do a screen test for a part in a TV pilot and had guaranteed him a lead in another TV pilot in the fall, if it was accepted. Not bad for a nine-year-old boy!

My thoughts were interrupted when I finally reached my destination and drove into the parking lot of Children's Hospital. As I entered the front door, I was directed to the oncology clinic on the first floor.

It is a frightening experience to find oneself in the oncology clinic. Gloria told me later that when she realized where she was and why she had been sent there, she made her way out to the reception area and cried out, "Oh God, not my son!" as she fainted and fell to the floor. She had to be revived by Michael's oncologist. Michael remained calm, trying to soothe his mother even though he, too, was beginning to suspect why he was there.

When I arrived, the waiting room of the clinic was filled with Michael's distraught relatives. Domenic's eyes were bloodshot from weeping. Michael's Italian grandparents, Armando and Anna; his two aunts, Rosa and Rena; his Uncle Steve and his Uncle Mike were totally downcast, praying silently from time to time. Gloria had been pacing the floor, waiting anxiously for the specialists' diagnosis. She couldn't wait any longer so she went to see how the specialists were progressing.

Michael came towards me looking composed, but his customary big smile was absent from his face. I wrapped my arms around him tightly, as if to shield him from his unknown adversary. I stepped back and looked down to where the two lumps around his collar bone were strongly evident.

"How long have you had those?" I asked. Surely we would have noticed them if they had been there for any length of time.

"Uncle Vince noticed them last week. My mom took me to Emergency that evening, and the doctor said that this was a result of infection from the strep throat I had been experiencing intermittently for six months. He prescribed more antibiotics and sent me home."

Michael further explained that, just this past weekend, he had been out on a paddle boat on Whonnock Lake with his friend, Brodie. It was a hot day so they had decided to jump into the water to cool themselves. When they tried to get back into the boat, Michael did not have the strength to do it. He passed out in the water. Luckily, Brodie jumped back into the water to help him. He kept Michael's head above the water until they reached the dock. Brodie shook him a few times and Michael revived. What a wonderful friend! They went to Brodie's mother, Shelley, and told her what had happened. When Gloria called to check to see how their day had gone, Shelley explained to Gloria what had taken place. She felt that

Michael might have mononucleosis instead of strep throat. Gloria was concerned and called her doctor. The doctor had examined Michael this morning and referred him to a specialist right away. The specialist then sent him to Children's Hospital for a second opinion, which resulted in his ending up in the oncology clinic. This all took place within a matter of hours.

"The specialists think that I could have mononucleosis, a viral infection, or cancer," Michael said matter-of-factly. He had insisted on being present during all discussions between his parents and the specialists.

This was so like Michael. He always made the best of bad situations. To him, they were problems that would be solved, satisfactorily, in time.

Suddenly, the two specialists appeared in the doorway. Our eyes scanned their faces for signs of the results of their findings regarding Michael's condition. The specialists suggested that Domenic and Gloria go into an adjoining room with them to discuss the matter. Michael insisted on going with them.

"What do you think, Jane?" Rosa asked me after they left.

"The news isn't going to be entirely good," I replied. I could tell by the looks on the specialists' faces. However, I did feel that things weren't completely hopeless either.

About 15 minutes later, Dr. Anderson reappeared with my daughter, son-in-law and grandson. Evidently, blood tests ruled out mononucleosis and a viral infection. Thankfully, leukemia was excluded also. A chest x-ray revealed shadowing in Michael's chest, which concerned the specialists. At this stage, their diagnosis suggested either Hodgkin's or Non-Hodgkin's lymphoma. Hodgkin's would be the lesser of the two evils.

Although Hodgkin's disease is believed to be a malignant lymph disease, it is more treatable, particularly if caught in its

early stages. The treatment usually involves chemotherapy and/or radiation. Non-Hodgkin's lymphoma is more dangerous because it spreads rapidly, so is less likely to be localized.

Tests conducted in the next few days will determine which type Michael has and whether it has spread to other parts of his body. There is so much at stake. The waiting seems endless.

While the others went home, I drove to the home of my grandchildren's Uncle Mike and Aunt Carla, who were looking after Sophia and Steven. It was Steven's birthday. Domenic and Gloria had planned on having all the family members over for the customary celebration. Due to the distressing turn of events, no one was in the mood for celebrating.

Even so, Carla had purchased a birthday cake for Steven. We sang "Happy Birthday" to him as he blew out the candles. Fortunately, his big party with his friends had been yesterday. Sophia, Steven, and I returned home about eight o'clock.

After Michael fell asleep watching TV, Gloria came downstairs to my suite and collapsed on the chesterfield. She sobbed agonizingly. I knew I was watching her experience the biggest heartbreak of her life. All I could do was hold her and weep silently with her as she cried, "God, please don't take my boy from me, I couldn't stand it."

I know that if she loses her son, I will not only lose my beloved grandson, but I will also lose my bubbly, vivacious daughter, who has always looked on life as an adventure. Nothing will ever be the same for us again.

 July 26, 1994

Before leaving with his mother, for the CT Scan (Computed Axial Tomography Scan) Michael provided us with a little comic relief. "First we prayed for mononucleosis or a viral infection; now we are praying for Hodgkin's disease," he observed dryly.

The CT Scan enables the radiologist to see and diagnose very small tumours that cannot be seen on ordinary x-rays. Tumours and other abnormalities in the soft tissues such as the brain, liver, pancreas, kidneys, bladder, adrenal glands, and pelvic organs can be spotted by a CT scan, also.

Although no tumours were found in the organs in Michael's body, a large mass of unexplained tissue was found around his heart and thymus. If this tissue was cancerous, there was a frightening possibility that the disease might have spread to his heart and lungs.

Domenic, Gloria, and Michael were informed by the specialists that Michael would require a biopsy of the lump on the right side of his collar bone.

Michael explained to the doctors that in two days he would be having a screen test for a part in a TV-series pilot. He requested that the biopsy be done as soon as possible, so he would be ready for the screen test.

The surgeon, Dr. Blair, postponed his vacation in order to perform a biopsy on Michael that evening. He said that he would leave as small a scar as possible, for which Michael was very thankful.

Since Domenic's father and mother live near the hospital, Domenic, Gloria, and Michael went there to rest and eat before returning to the hospital for the operation.

Michael's grandparents, aunts, and uncles came to the hospital while Michael was having his surgery. Michael had been given some medication to help him relax in preparation for the biopsy. This medication, and the procedure he was facing, made Michael very emotional. He wanted to talk to his relatives, in couples, before he was taken away for surgery. Michael asked each couple to pray for him, and said he loved them. He kept saying, "It's not cancer, it's just a virus. I'll be all right." He was still hoping that he didn't have cancer. After leaving Michael, everybody had tears in their eyes as they silently prayed for a miracle.

Following the surgery, the surgeon who had done the biopsy spoke with Domenic and Gloria. He explained that a section was removed from the lump for an immediate microscopic examination by a pathologist. This preliminary test is not infallible, but it is a strong indicator as to whether the area is malignant or not. Although the surgeon is fairly certain that Michael was suffering from Hodgkin's disease, final confirmation will come tomorrow. The doctors explained Hodgkin's disease to us.

It is divided into categories A and B, based on whether a person has certain symptoms. The disease can progress from painless swelling of the lymph glands to the more advanced B symptoms, which include abdominal discomfort due to an enlarged spleen, loss of more than 10 percent of body weight in the previous six months, fever without any known cause, night sweats, and weakness.

Hodgkin's is further divided into four stages:

Stage 1 Cancer
is found in only one lymph node area or in only one area or organ outside of the lymph nodes.

Stage 2 Cancer
is found in two or more lymph node areas on the same side of the diaphragm. Cancer is found in only one area or organ outside of the lymph nodes and in the lymph nodes around it.

Stage 3 Cancer
> *is found in lymph node areas on both sides of the diaphragm. The cancer may also have spread to an area or organ near the lymph node areas or to the spleen.*

Stage 4 Cancer
> *has spread in more than one spot to an organ or organs outside the lymph system. Cancer cells may or may not be found in the lymph nodes near these organs.*

A Gallium test is used to determine the spread of the disease. This test involves injecting a very tiny amount of radioactive Gallium into the body. Over the next two days, the radioactive substance circulates throughout the body. The Gallium localizes at sites where a disease such as lymphoma may be present. The patient then undergoes a nuclear medicine scan of the entire body to detect whether or not there is a localization of Gallium in certain parts of the body. If there is, a malignancy is a strong possibility.

 July 27, 1994

The final results of the biopsy have confirmed that Michael has Hodgkin's disease. All hopes of there being some mistake have vanished. We have no choice; we have to accept the fact that Michael has cancer.

Michael has been allowed to come home today.

 July 28, 1994

Gloria took Michael for a screen test for a TV-series pilot. He decided not to mention anything about having Hodgkin's disease to the director. He wasn't wanting to be deceitful—he just didn't want his having the disease to affect the director's decision. I wonder what the director would think if he knew about the real life drama Michael is experiencing. It far surpasses any part he could play on the screen.

July 30, 1994

Michael received the good news today that he has been chosen for the pilot. He's also been told that if the pilot is picked up, he is assured a lead role in the series.

Later on, when the producers found out that Michael had Hodgkin's, they were very understanding. They allowed him to wear either a bandanna or hat to cover up his hair loss.

 Aug. 1, 1994

Domenic and Gloria took Michael to the hospital to receive an injection of radioactive Gallium. Michael came home with them, but will have to go back to the hospital for the scan in two days.

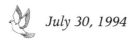 *Aug. 3, 1994*

Michael was readmitted to Children's Hospital for bone marrow tests and to have a Vascular Access Device (VAD) inserted under the skin. In Michael's case, it was inserted below the left side of his collar bone. Instead of having a needle in his arm every time he needed blood tests or medicine, the connections could be made through the tubing extending from the VAD, making these procedures much less painful.

We had some good news. Michael's bone marrow tests reveal no cancer in the bone marrow. However, when they completed the Gallium test, it revealed that the cancer had spread throughout his chest, including into the thymus and outside the heart region. This is cause for great concern.

Michael's Hodgkin's disease was classified as 2A, since he didn't have any B symptoms. Treatment of Hodgkin's disease involves chemotherapy, radiation and sometimes total nodal eradication. Michael is starting off with chemotherapy. Since he is under ten years of age, radiation, if needed, will be used sparingly to avoid retarding his growth. Right now, the outlook for Michael's future is uncertain, to say the least. We will not let ourselves think of Michael not surviving. We can't bear to think of that possibility.

Statistics currently show that five years cancer-free, Michael's survival rate will be 75 to 85 percent. Ten years cancer-free, his survival rate goes up to 90 percent.

Michael had three things going for him which would increase his chances for survival. Being a firm believer in the power of prayer, I will put it first. All of Michael's relatives and friends, as well as my church and Gloria and Domenic's church, were praying for him. Secondly, Michael was receiving excellent medical care. Thirdly, Michael has a positive attitude towards life that gave him the determination to live.

I can think of at least four times, in the next two years, when Michael's survival was simply miraculous.

Chapter 2

The Treatments Begin

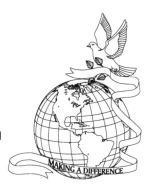

 Aug. 6, 1994

Today Michael was admitted to Ward 3B of Children's Hospital for his first round of chemotherapy treatments. He will be in the hospital for a few days because it is essential that he be monitored closely to ensure that his body is able to tolerate the chemotherapy drugs that have been prescribed for him. The protocol will need to be changed if the combination of drugs are interacting unfavourably, subjecting Michael to dangerous side effects.

Michael is saddened when he hears the cries of so many children suffering from cancer. He is sharing a room with a little boy who was diagnosed with cancer at five months old. The little boy is having a VAD inserted into his chest for further chemotherapy treatments. What a way to celebrate his first birthday! Michael had been given some balloons, and he gave these to the boy as a birthday present. Michael is shocked that children can get cancer so young.

Michael's chemotherapy treatments are scheduled to last for a total of six months. His treatment protocol will be consistent each month. In Week One he will start taking chemotherapy pills every day. One day out of Week Two will be spent as an out-patient at the oncology clinic receiving chemotherapy through his VAD. Chemotherapy takes eight to ten days to take effect, and it is then that the patient has a "bad week."

Michael experienced severe nausea, hot and cold spells, dizziness, headaches and tiredness during this time.

During the two weeks Michael is on chemotherapy, he is to take one Septra pill daily, Monday to Wednesday, to prevent lung infection; two chemotherapy pills daily for a week; and one and a half Ondonsatron pills, to relieve nausea, one hour before the chemotherapy pills. He is also to take one and a half Prednisone pills, daily, for six months. The Prednisone will give him an appetite and keep him from losing weight.

In some ways, it was like living on the edge of a volcano. The situation seemed reasonably calm, but there was always the possibility that the side effects of the drugs Michael had to take could erupt and devastate us all with their serious consequences. We were on guard, constantly watching for any of these symptoms in Michael.

The chemotherapy drugs have great risks. The names of these drugs and their side effects are outlined as follows:

Adriamycin

Causes red stained urine, interferes with the production of blood cells, can cause blood clotting disorders, anemia and infections. Blood counts must be carefully monitored. Hair loss common. Dose dependent changes in heart rhythm and heart failure are risks.

Monitoring: checks on blood composition, regular heart examinations and liver function tests.

Bleomycin

Same risks and monitoring as for Adriamycin.

Cyclophosphamide

Causes nausea and hair loss. It can affect the heart, liver, and bladder. Often reduces blood cell production so can lead to abnormal bleeding, increased risk of infection and reduced fertility in men.

Monitoring: periodic checks on blood composition and all the effects of the drug.

Procarbazine
Nausea, anemia and blood clotting disorders, susceptibility to rises in blood pressure, damage to the central nervous system with numbness of hands and feet, unsteadiness, headache, depression, nightmares, tremors and confusion.

Monitoring: periodic blood tests.

Vinblastine
Headache, jaw pain, difficulty walking, difficulty urinating, tingling and numbness in hands and feet, constipation, swelling of tongue, hoarse voice and sore throat.

Vincristine
Difficulty walking, difficulty urinating, tingling and numbness in hands and feet, jaw pain, double vision and constipation.

It was Michael's stalwart acceptance of his cancer that gave the rest of the family the strength to rally and get through the next six months. Wisely, he made up his mind to keep up his normal activities when he was symptom-free from the drugs he was taking. He rode with wild abandon the new 21-speed bicycle his parents bought him. He roller-bladed and skate-boarded as usual. He was unable to do any swimming because of the VAD inserted in his chest. He particularly missed being able to do this activity, since it was still summer.

At a one-week day camp, he kept up with the rest of the children in their activities. He went on all the rides at the Pacific National Exhibition. He joined in all the races at the annual Italian picnic and danced up a storm at their evening dance. At this event, he performed the song *One Moment In Time*, which had words very pertinent to his situation before his cancer: *"Give me one moment in time, when I'm racing with destiny, when all of my dreams are a heartbeat away, and the answers are all up to me."* Little did he know then that he was racing with destiny.

Chapter 3

Back To School

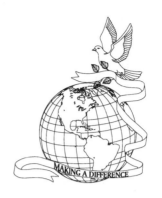

 August 1994

Often, when one child in a family becomes seriously ill, there is a concern that the other children can feel neglected. After their initial compassion for their ill sibling, resentment towards the time spent on this child, and the special treatment that the child receives, can start to emerge.

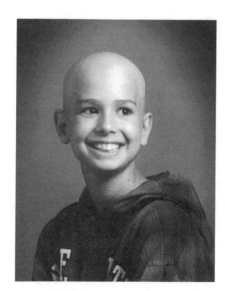

Michael's grade four school photograph (9 ½ yrs).

"I can't understand Sophia," Gloria lamented earlier today. "Michael's been sick a month. Why doesn't she groom herself, straighten her room, or help me around the house?"

"I think I know what's bothering her," I said. "Her friends are away at a day camp and she is missing out because you've been so caught up with Michael that you didn't get her registered."

"I know. I have been so absorbed with what has happened to him, I never got around to doing it. I'll see if I can get her into the last week of camp."

 Aug. 15 - 19, 1994

Gloria was able to enroll all three children at day camp. They are having a great time rock-climbing, cliff-jumping and roller-skating with their friends. They also enjoyed a tour of Britannia Mines and did some panning for gold. Michael felt well at camp, and didn't experience any problems in keeping up with his group.

In preparation for the start of a new school year, Gloria took Sophia shopping for some new clothes and treated her to a visit to the hairdresser. Her conscious effort to spend a little more time with Sophia has resulted in a noticeable improvement in Sophia's attitude. She has become more amiable with those around her and she is helping out more around the house. Relations between mother and daughter have improved considerably.

These circumstances with Sophia have prompted Domenic and Gloria to consider how Michael's disease is affecting the whole family. Although Sophia is older and receives a lot of support from her friends, she still needs time spent with her mom and dad. Steven, accustomed to spending a lot of one-on-one time with Gloria, is just about to start attending school full-time. Domenic and Gloria were striving to provide support for all of their children, which is a difficult balance to achieve at this time. Gloria had been running a home-party fashion-wear business for several years. As much as she had enjoyed this pursuit, she has now decided to give it up so she can devote more time to her family.

Domenic and Gloria also took time to talk with the children. It was explained to Sophia and Steven what help would be needed during the months ahead. One of Gloria's suggestions was that they could each pray for Michael's recovery. Steven liked to join Gloria in prayer each night, while Sophia preferred to pray on her own.

It was comforting to Domenic and Gloria to know that I was at home for Sophia and Steven when they needed me. I did my best to nurture my grandchildren as much as possible. Often, I would take them to their after-school activities or help them with their homework. I took Sophia and Steven to swimming lessons. Other times I stayed at the pool with Steven while he swam with his friends. Domenic and Gloria enrolled him in roller-blade hockey. Between his parents and me, someone always attended his games.

Domenic was able to continue to carry out his work responsibilities because of the knowledge that the situation at home was under control. Additionally, Michael's own strength in coping with his cancer helped the family immensely.

 Aug. 30, 1994

What we have been worrying about in connection with Michael's chemotherapy treatments has happened sooner than we had anticipated. Michael's tawny brown hair has started to fall out. School is only a week away. We are wondering how Michael will respond. Will his classmates make fun of him? Will his auditions for commercials and movies cease?

Gloria decided to take Michael and Steven to the hairdresser. Steven had his hair cut in his usual style, shaved at the bottom and long at the top.

Michael sat down in the chair next to Steven. "Do you want your hair cut in the same style, Michael?" the hairdresser asked.

"I want it shaved off," Michael replied.

"You mean a buzz cut."

"No, I want it all shaved off."

The hairdresser looked at Gloria dubiously. My daughter nodded her assent. Reluctantly, the hairdresser proceeded to fulfill Michael's request.

When the procedure was over, Michael looked in the mirror and beamed. He liked the haircut, or I should say, shave. His sister, Sophia, paid a compliment to Michael when she proclaimed his hairstyle "rad."

I must say that Michael looks better than I thought he would. He has been blessed with a well-shaped head and ears that are reasonable in size. He feels that he will draw less attention to himself at school if he starts without hair, rather than have it fall out after school begins.

 Sept. 6, 1994

Today was the first day of school for my three grandchildren, in grades one, four, and seven. Domenic, Gloria, and I were particularly concerned that Michael would be teased about not having any hair. Sure enough, it has already happened. When Michael was out in the playground, some boys started calling Michael "Baldy," "Skin Head," "Geek," "Retard," "Poor Baby."

Other children, hearing the name-calling, went to the office and reported the matter to the principal. He came out and read the riot act to the boys: "This boy is going through a hard time right now and he is being strong about it. If you boys ever do this again, you are out of this school."

He took Michael to one side and told him that if anyone did this again they would be suspended from school. This principal has very few discipline problems in his school because he always deals with these kinds of problems firmly and promptly. We are so pleased he is supporting Michael.

 Sept. 7, 1994

Michael had his own ideas about how he was going to deal with his hair situation. Today, working in pairs, the class was doing a worksheet on their likes and dislikes. Michael and his partner came to the part where they chose their favourite entertainer. Michael chose Christina Applegate.

"Have you looked in the mirror lately? You wouldn't have a chance with her, baldy," his partner said.

"Trust me, you'll never get to be a comedian," Michael retorted.

"Looks like there is some steam coming out of those little hairs," ventured his partner.

A smack echoed throughout the room as Michael handled the problem his way. "Next time, it will be my fist, not my hand," Michael said menacingly.

The teacher demonstrated support for Michael in a number of ways. She asked Michael's partner to leave the room to contemplate Michael's situation. While she understood Michael's angry response, she also gave him the means to prevent future problems. From then on he was allowed to wear a hat in class. He seems quite comfortable with this solution.

 Sept. 8, 1994

Michael, in general, is handling his baldness quite well. He is even developing a sense of humour where his baldness is concerned. At the Canadian Pacific Railway picnic Michael sang karaoke. "Whom are you dedicating this song to?" one man asked.

"My bald-headed dad," Michael said, pointing to his father.

"He's not bald—look at me," the man said, pointing to his practically bald head.

Michael snatched off his own Penguins hat and exclaimed, "I'm the baldest of all of you."

Chapter 4

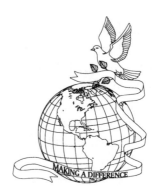

Experiencing Drug Side Effects

 Sept. 9, 1994

Michael's second set of chemotherapy treatments started today. He also went for pulmonary tests, a cardiogram, and x-rays. These measures would determine whether the drugs were affecting his heart and lungs adversely, and if the drugs were shrinking the mass of cancer in his chest. There was good news. The test results are reassuring in all respects.

 Sept. 12, 1994

Michael keeps asking his mother to let him use his skate board. This has been a concern for Gloria. Today she finally relented. Little did she know that he was planning to go down a nearby hill which is extremely steep. When he was doing so, he took a very bad fall, scraping his elbow and taking a patch of skin off his waist. Gloria became upset and worried that he could hemorrhage or get a severe infection. It's hard not to worry when his blood platelet count is so low and his resistance is weak.

 Sept. 14, 1994

Michael is experiencing a side effect from the drug Prednisone. It has been making him feel easily frustrated. When Michael was working on his homework, including a reading assignment which is due in a week, he temporarily lost control. "I am so frustrated, I feel like breaking everything in the house!" he yelled. "I want to feel normal again and I want my hair back!"

"Go ahead and let it out," I said. "You have been so brave since this has happened, it will do you good. Too bad you don't have a punching bag."

Gloria came downstairs to see what the commotion was about and said, "You can't demolish the house even if you are frustrated." I told her that Michael's pent-up emotions needed some kind of release.

"I will take you to the golf range and you can hit a few balls. It will help you to get rid of some of your frustration," Gloria said.

Michael brightened considerably. They returned home about an hour later looking relaxed. My grandson was also pleased that his mother had agreed to let him join soccer. He was eager to participate in sports activities.

 Sept. 16, 1994

Michael seems very anxious to appear "normal." Even though it is his "bad week," he's playing soccer. Today, Michael kept body checking one of the boys to keep him from scoring. The boy retaliated by making fun of Michael's bald head. This angered Michael to the point where he pushed the boy. They both ended up being yellow-carded. Another yellow card and Michael would have been out of the game.

Seeing that Michael was upset, the coach said, "Get even— go and score a goal. That will fix him." In the next few minutes Michael did just that, as well as receiving an assist. While the game was still going on, Michael raced to some bushes where he became violently ill. He then rejoined the game as if nothing had happened. His team did end up winning the game.

Michael is continuing to participate in a variety of other activities. He and his friend Brodie are involved in jazz dance lessons together and have recently placed first in a dance competition. We were all very proud and happy for them. The choreography required physical strength and agility, which Michael was able to summon, despite having just finished his "bad week" of chemotherapy.

Domenic has purchased a keyboard for Michael and he has started taking piano lessons. The piano teacher is amazed at Michael's natural musical ability. Michael has even begun to dabble with composing a tune. Life is more settled within our household than it has been since Michael was diagnosed. Gloria is planning a surprise 40th birthday party for Domenic, which is scheduled for New Year's Eve.

 Oct. 8, 1994

Domenic's mother, Anna, and Sophia were both born on October 11th. Sophia celebrated her 12th birthday today with friends. Domenic and Gloria rented a Space Ball Ride for the party. This unique and exciting amusement ride was a great hit. Sophia hosted a birthday dinner and a sleep-over for her friends. Everyone had fun and it was a wonderfully lighthearted day.

 Oct. 9, 1994

All the family gathered at Domenic's parents house to celebrate a family birthday for Anna and Sophia. We also shared a nice Thanksgiving meal. We had a joyous day together.

 Oct. 27, 1994

Gloria told me today that she was feeling somewhat reluctant to carry on with making the plans for Domenic's December 31st surprise party. Michael is encouraging her to go ahead with the party plans. He really seems to be anticipating the event. No doubt it is giving him something to look forward to.

Unbelievably, before the plans for the December party could be finalized, Michael was to face another great calamity in his life.

 Oct. 31, 1994

Today was Halloween and it was also Michael's three month appointment at Children's Hospital. A born entertainer, he dressed up for his visit to the oncology clinic. His bald head was covered with a long curly red wig he had borrowed from Brodie's mother. Michael had worn one of Gloria's dresses. It was tight-fitting, black, and stuffed with padding in the appropriate places.

When Gloria and Michael returned home they had fantastic news. Dr. Anderson told them today that Michael's chest x-rays were clear. There were no visible signs of cancer and this indicated that the chemotherapy was working. We felt very encouraged.

Still in costume, Michael went on to share stories about the fun he had making people laugh. His unforgettable summary was, "What makes me happiest in life is when I make other people happy."

Although the x-rays showed that Michael's chest was clear of cancer, there was always the possibility that minute cells, not visible on the x-rays, remained. In a situation such as this, the team of oncologists often have to determine whether the patient's treatment should be continued or not. Each form of treatment for cancer carries its own dangers. The side effects and risks of the treatment must be weighed against the risk of the cancer returning if treatment is discontinued. Dr. Anderson and the rest of the specialists would soon be meeting to discuss the treatment plan for Michael.

Chapter 5

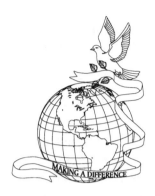

Another Nightmare

 Nov. 14, 1994

Michael is in his fourth month of chemotherapy. Tonight, while Michael was working on his homework, he started to complain about a terrible headache. This is the "bad" week when the drugs take effect, so we think that he might be having a toxic headache. He went to bed, but he didn't sleep. Severe nausea and vomiting have started. What now?

 Nov. 15, 1994

Michael's symptoms have worsened since yesterday. When his temperature reached 103°F, Gloria called Dr. Anderson, who told her to bring Michael into Children's Hospital immediately. During the one hour drive to the hospital, Michael was still vomiting and experiencing severe head pain. He was rushed to the oncology clinic upon arrival.

Michael's blood pressure was fluctuating constantly as a result of severe dehydration. While fluids were steadily administered to Michael by intravenous, the specialists began performing a series of tests. The doctors did everything they could to stabilize his condition. There was a nurse monitoring Michael at all times. Domenic and Gloria stayed at his side. Throughout this ordeal, Michael remained calm and insisted that he was going to be all right.

Dr. Anderson suspected infection so one of the tests ordered was a spinal tap. This test would confirm if Michael had meningitis, and whether it was viral or bacterial. Within an hour, the doctors informed us that Michael had indeed contracted meningitis.

The news was devastating. Overwhelmed by emotion, Gloria went to a private room, where she broke down in tears. She was terrified that she was going to lose her son. Domenic

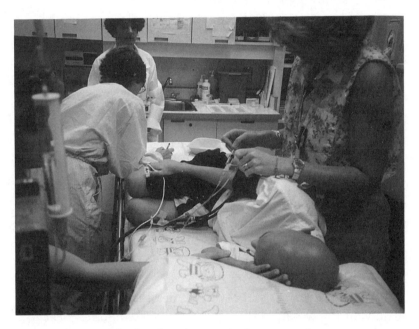

*Michael undergoing a spinal tap procedure
to determine if he has meningitis.*

held his emotions inside, staying with Michael until Gloria was able to rejoin them. The next 48 hours would determine what course the disease would take. All Domenic and Gloria could do was wait and watch their son suffer. How much more are they going to be able to stand?

Although we wracked our brains later at home, it remained a mystery how Michael had caught such a terrible disease. All we could fathom was that his immune system had been suppressed due to the chemotherapy treatments.

 Nov. 18, 1994

Michael has miraculously rallied during the past 48 hours. The infectious control team from Children's Hospital has not been able to determine for certain whether Michael's meningitis is viral or bacterial. Therefore, Michael must stay in an isolation room at the hospital for ten days.

Gloria has been at the hospital for three days straight. Domenic goes to the hospital every night after dinner, periodically bringing Sophia and Steven to visit Michael.

Staying in the hospital, in one room, never being allowed to set foot outside of the door, Michael has become restless. To relieve the monotony, he asked Domenic to bring his keyboard to the hospital. Unbeknownst to us, while Michael was in isolation he wrote the lyrics to the song for his father's fortieth birthday party. Evidently, a melody and beat had been going through his mind for some time. The words he wrote expressed how he missed his father when Domenic was working and couldn't be with Michael in the hospital. He was also thinking of children who had passed away from this disease and how he missed them after they were gone. Thus, his first song, *When You Are Away*, came into being.

With the latest crisis in Michael's health, Gloria was once again wanting to cancel the party. Michael would not hear of it. It has become apparent to Gloria that the thought of the party was providing Michael with the inner strength that he needed to cope with his illnesses.

Michael has been maintaining a brave front to avoid upsetting his family. This is so like him. He always looks for a silver lining behind each cloud. I've begun to wonder where the silver linings are for Michael. He's been blessed with so much

talent, but his luck seems to be extremely poor. Just as things start going well for him, something else hits. Through it all, he grins, jokes, and assesses the situation with amazing optimism. Everyone who meets him feels that they have come in contact with a very special person. Why is God allowing him to be tested to this extent? Hasn't he passed all his tests with flying colours? When will he reap some rewards?

 Nov. 28, 1994

Michael came home today. He's looking great considering what he has been through. It is wonderful to have him back with us!

Chapter 6

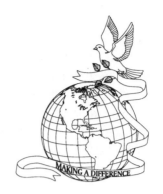

We Celebrate

 Dec. 10, 1994

Good news about Michael! The best Christmas present for all of us! Michael's CT scan and Gallium tests show that he is completely cancer-free. His oncologist has told Domenic and Gloria that Michael will not need his sixth regimen of chemotherapy treatments. What a miracle! We have another big reason to celebrate.

 Dec. 31, 1994

Gloria deliberately planned the birthday party for New Year's Eve, so Domenic would be fooled as to the real reason behind this celebration. The party turned out to be a great success. All our friends and relatives attended.

Michael was master of ceremonies and proved to be a natural. He was a fantastic stand-up comedian. His one-liners were hilarious.

The Cuccione men lose their hair early in life. Michael bragged that he was now a member of the Cuccione Bald-Headed Club. The only difference, he went on, was that he would get his hair back!

When Michael sang *When You Are Away* and dedicated it to his father, there wasn't a dry eye in the place. This was one of the few times that Michael had seen his father cry.

Domenic had shed many tears over Michael's situation, but he tried not to let Michael see them.

Each guest received a scroll containing the words of the song and Michael presented a framed copy of the song to his father. When Domenic came up to receive his gift, he hugged Michael warmly. He was so overcome with emotion that he could scarcely speak. He expressed his gratitude to Michael for this gift and added that the greatest gift of all was the fact that Michael was cancer-free.

 Jan. 28, 1995

We've been waiting for the radiologist's decision as to whether or not Michael requires radiation to ensure the fact he remains cancer-free. Dr. Anderson called Gloria with the verdict. Michael will not receive radiation because it could damage his heart and lungs. We are relieved. They will need to give Michael his sixth regimen of chemotherapy instead. How on earth can we break this news to Michael?

Domenic and Gloria explained the situation to Michael as carefully as they could. He burst into tears and was extremely upset. It was like reliving a nightmare to him. He had thought that his ordeal was over, but now he has to face more chemotherapy. His hair is starting to grow back and he will lose it again. Michael observed, "If this disease is going to come back, it won't make any difference if I have five *or* six treatments." Domenic and Gloria explained their views.

Michael grudgingly has agreed that he will go ahead with the treatment. In Domenic and Gloria's minds, they could never forgive themselves if Michael's disease came back because he hadn't had his sixth treatment.

After Michael recovered from his last chemotherapy treatment he started working on his second song, Make a Difference. *He was determined that he was going to try to make*

a difference by helping to put an end to the pain and suffering of cancer.

We were amazed at this new talent of Michael's. We knew that he was gifted in singing, dancing, and acting, but we had no idea that he could write lyrics.

Domenic and Gloria decided to give Michael voice lessons in addition to his piano lessons. They also enlisted the services of Terry Robotham, a fantastic musician, to help Michael to record his songs. The goal was for Michael to compose three more songs and record them on a CD, with net proceeds going to cancer research. Michael would come up with the chords on his keyboard, and would sing his songs onto a tape. Terry would use the tape to help do the background music. The music would be then put onto a demo tape, allowing Michael to perform at functions and to practise in preparation for recording the songs. Michael spent a lot of time in the recording studio. Even when he wasn't feeling well, he would stay focused on his goals throughout the coming months.

 Mar. 6, 1995

Michael is having his three-month checkup. We got another scare. The CT scan, pulmonary function and ECG (electrocardiogram) tests turned out fine, but the Gallium test shows a take-up of Gallium around the tissue of his thymus, the site of his original cancer. We're in shock. There is a possibility that Michael's cancer has not been completely cured. How will Michael be able to deal with the return of his cancer? How will we be able to cope? Two of the cancer patients with whom Michael had played Nintendo have already died.

 Mar. 9, 1995

We're relieved. The specialists told us that it was natural for the thymus to be swollen—it was just the result of his body fighting off the cancer and the effects of the drugs that he has been taking. They call it thymus rebound. They don't believe that the cancer has returned. We can only hope that they are right. Three months from now we will have to go through the same thing again, and again for the next five or ten years. It is becoming a constant fear lurking in the back of our minds.

How do you deal with this kind of fear? We believe that the answer is to go on with life as normally as possible. That is what Michael is doing and is encouraging others to do the same.

Even when he is going through his chemotherapy treatments, he keeps on with most of his usual activities. He is missing very little schooling. He seizes every moment of life for what it is worth, whether the remaining time left to him be long or short. You can see that he is not going to die within himself, long before his physical death.

 Apr. 15, 1995

The family has just returned from their trip to Disneyland in California. Michael is particularly eager to pursue his musical goals. Michael's first chance to perform his songs came at the Miss Calabria Pageant, a major Italian event. He sang *Make a Difference* and told the audience about his dream to produce a CD to help fight cancer. One of the coordinators of the program handed a box to Michael, placed $100 in it, and challenged others to follow his example. In a matter of minutes, about $1,100 was raised to further Michael's dream.

 May 10, 1995

Michael was interviewed on a multicultural program promoting the Italian telethon for B.C.'s Children's Hospital, which will be televised May 26 and 27. He was interviewed by Anna Terrana. She told Michael that he wears his soul in his eyes. Michael sang *Make a Difference* again. He was so relaxed and natural that you would think that he was conducting the interview from his living room. He even ended the interview with a bit of Italian that he had picked up from his relatives.

When Michael was asked about his future career plans he took a deep breath and said, "I want to work hard to help find a cure for cancer. I want to stop the pain and the dying. I want to make a difference." It was easy for Michael to answer that question. This is how he feels. The answer came straight from his heart.

 May 12, 1995

Michael told his mother that he is feeling like his old self again. He is certainly looking well. He has lots of energy, is eating well and is happy that his hair is coming back. Michael and the others are really looking forward to the summer holidays and have many exciting plans ahead. They are determined to make up for the times they missed during the previous summer.

 May 15, 1995

Michael has been excitedly preparing for his school track and field events. He has spent many days practising for high jump, the 100 metre race and 400 metre race, the shot put, long jump, and the medley relay. Today was the day of the meet and Michael managed to place in all events.

The medley relay was a triumph for Michael. In the relay there are four racers on each team. The first racer runs 400 metres. The baton is then passed to the next racer, who runs 100 metres. That person passes it to the next person who runs 100 metres as well. That person passed the baton to Michael, who ran the last 200 metres. Michael was able to bring his team from fourth place to second place!

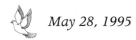 *May 28, 1995*

Michael performed live on the Italian telethon .The proceeds from the telethon will be donated to B.C.'s Children's Hospital.

Michael has also been invited to be a part of the main telethon for B.C.'s Children's Hospital, which airs live on UTV next week-end. He will be presenting the $1,100 to Children's Hospital, and is going to be filmed singing *Make a Difference.* Michael's dream has gotten off to a great start!

Chapter 7

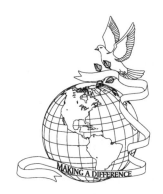

What Do We Do Now?

 June 20, 1995

Michael had his three-month follow-up appointment. The blood tests results were fine. Dr. Anderson was very pleased, but he did ask Michael to take a routine chest x-ray before leaving the hospital.

 June 21, 1995

Gloria received an alarming phone call from Dr. Anderson today . He told her that he was concerned about some shadowing that had shown up on the x-rays of Michael's chest. Dr. Anderson requested more x-rays be taken. Gloria is sick about this. She tried to down play the situation with Michael but he seemed confused and wondered what was happening.

 June 23, 1995

Domenic, Gloria, and Michael went to Children's Hospital this afternoon to have the other set of x-rays taken.

Dr. Anderson and a nurse called the three of them into a private room in the oncology clinic. Dr. Anderson explained that the x-rays had shown spots on Michael's lungs and there were shadows above and below his heart. More Gallium tests and another CT Scan will be required to determine specifically what was going on. With tears in his eyes, Dr. Anderson had to tell them that the cancer has returned and has spread to both lungs.

Michael responded to this news with a combination of anger and resignation: "What are my chances now? Am I terminal?"

Domenic put his head down to keep from fainting. Gloria reacted with denial: "This can't be, how can we be sure? He has been feeling so good lately! It must be a chest infection of some sort."

Dr. Anderson could truly understand their anguish. He assured Michael that he was not terminal, but he would need heavy chemotherapy and a bone marrow transplant to treat the disease. Dr. Anderson said that he had faith in Michael and was sure that one day he would be enjoying a normal life again.

Domenic, Gloria, and Michael returned home and tried to come to grips with the devastating news. Michael called his friend Chris, and went over to his house for a while to try to forget what had happened. Michael shared this news with his friend, who reacted with total disbelief.

We decided to downplay the news to Sophia and Steven until we were completely certain that these results are accurate. Afterwards, Sophia and Steven wanted to go visit their cousins. Domenic, Gloria, and I took advantage of the time without the children to deal with our emotions. I felt like I had been struck by lightning. We were all overcome by shock at what Michael was facing, and so frustrated because there was nothing we could do about it.

Domenic phoned his family and gave them the terrible news. They came over right away. They did their best to comfort us but we were numb. There was little that could be said that would really reach us.

Gloria spent most of the evening in her room crying. *She said later that she had learned what it was like to experience a true broken heart.*

Later that evening Domenic's relatives left, and the children returned home. We tried to lighten up for Michael's sake. We each went to our beds hoping and praying that this diagnosis would not be confirmed.

 June 24 & 25, 1995

We spent the weekend in a state of shock. None of us wanted to accept the possibility of a return of Michael's cancer! We hoped it would be an infection of some sort, or perhaps tuberculosis.

Maybe we should try alternate treatments. I've read about Billy Best. He fled from his home in Norwell, Massachusetts, rather than have any more chemotherapy for his Hodgkin's. He agreed to return home if he could try a revolutionary new treatment for cancer called 714X, a compound made from camphor, nitrogen and organic salts. He was also going to drink Essiac tea daily. According to Dr. Cliff Takemoto of Boston's Dan-Forber Cancer Institute, Billy is presently cancer-free. Maybe we could try these.

 June 26, 1995

Over the weekend, Dr. Anderson couldn't stop thinking about what Gloria had said about Michael possibly suffering from a lung infection. Just to make sure that this is not the case, he felt that Michael should have a biopsy.

Today, Michael had his bone marrow tested to determine if it is free of cancer cells. This is a very painful procedure. Michael needed medication to deal with his pain. Groggily, he muttered, "Why am I having to go through this again ?" There is no answer to this question. He has had one lucky break—there are no cancer cells in his bone marrow.

 June 27, 1995

Michael went in for his biopsy. At 8 a.m. the surgeon inserted a tube through Michael's trachea to the thymus region. Initially no cancer was found and Michael was sent to the recovery room. However, the doctor wanted to retrieve more tissue so a second biopsy was performed around noon. It was decided to go in through Michael's chest, where his VAD had previously been inserted. This was very dangerous because the surgery involved working over Michael's heart. The second pathology results that came back still showed no evidence of cancer.

Domenic and Gloria thought they were experiencing a miracle. At this time they were allowed to go to the recovery room to see Michael. When he opened his eyes, his first words were, "Is the cancer back?" He was so relieved when his parents said that it wasn't, he fell back to sleep.

As Domenic and Gloria turned to leave the recovery room, they met a nurse and Dr. Anderson. He wanted to discuss the next step so they all went into a room. The heart specialist also joined them. Dr. Anderson explained that because the x-rays and CT Scan had strongly indicated the disease was back, they wanted to perform yet a third biopsy. They planned to go in yet again through the same incision where the VAD had been. Each time another surgery is performed, Domenic's or Gloria's consent is required. Since Gloria could not bear to see her son suffer anymore, she left the decision up to Domenic. He felt that they had no other choice; they would have to go over Michael's heart one more time.

Dr. Anderson felt that Domenic had made the right choice. The operation was performed. Four pieces of tissue were removed and a pathologist did an on-spot freeze test. Tragically, this time the preliminary biopsy results confirmed that the cancer was back.

When Michael awakened, Domenic and Gloria had to break this terrible news to him. He was still so groggy from the effects of the anesthetic it is doubtful that the full implication of the biopsy registered with him at this time.

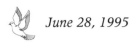 *June 28, 1995*

Michael is still in the hospital recovering from his biopsies. Final reports have confirmed that Michael's cancer is back and has spread to his lungs! A bone marrow is a must.

Dr. Anderson and several of his colleagues met with Domenic, Gloria, and Michael today. They discussed at length the procedures that will be involved in Michael's bone marrow transplant.

Dr. Anderson then outlined the risks involved, which are many. There could be life-threatening infections (bacterial, viral or fungal). Since Michael's bone marrow will be destroyed by the chemotherapy, he was at risk for hemorrhaging and mouth sores may occur, requiring morphine for the pain. The chemotherapy drugs could induce heart failure, decrease lung function, or cause shut-down of any other major organs.

Domenic, Gloria, and Michael feel they don't have much choice other than to go ahead with the transplant.
Dr. Anderson invited Michael to express his feelings about the procedure. Michael very bravely responded, "We have to just go for it." Dr. Anderson was amazed at the maturity Michael was showing about what lies ahead for him.

It is a nightmare! We can't believe that this is happening!

In the type of Bone Marrow Transplant that Michael will undergo, a central line hook-up is used for retrieving bone marrow stem cells and for administering the chemotherapy treatments. The patient initially receives high doses of chemotherapy to destroy the cancer cells in the body. Following that, Granulocyte-Colony Stimulating Factor(G-CSF) is injected under the skin of either the patient's arms or legs. This stimulates the bone marrow to push newly formed stem cells into the peripheral blood. From there, the new stem cells are

harvested, via a large bore catheter, with the use of a pheresis machine. These stem cells are stored in a frozen state until they are required for 'rescuing' the patient during the actual transplant. Then a second session of heavy chemotherapy is administered to destroy the existent bone marrow. The patient is then 'rescued' with the stem cells that were previously collected.

Despite the news, Michael is determined to leave the hospital in order to attend his sister Sophia's grade seven graduation tomorrow. He also wants to say good-bye to everyone at his school. Michael has missed being in the talent show today. The principal said that Michael can be interviewed by the local press and have his song, *Make a Difference*, played at the end of the assembly. Michael is unable to sing due to the effects of the biopsies. However, he will be speaking to everyone at his school.

 June 29, 1995

Michael managed to make an appearance at the grade seven graduation today. How he did it, I'll never know. He was so weak that he was barely able to walk to the front of the room to deliver his speech. He spoke of his goal of completing five songs and producing a CD. He wants the net proceeds from the sale of these CDs to be used for cancer research.

He said that he was determined to make a difference, but he wanted everyone to help so that a *really big* difference could be made. He wished the grade sevens a great time in high school and a bright future. His voice trembled here. He knew that not only would he be losing another summer, but that he was also facing the biggest fight of his life.

Wearing his No Fear T-shirt, clutching the microphone in his right hand, Michael raised two fingers symbolizing his second battle with cancer. His determination to overcome this

Message *from* Michael

By Maria Antonia Marano
Metro Valley News Service

"One person can only do so much, but together we can do much more. And I'm not leaving: there's much to do."

On June 27, Michael Cuccione, 10, underwent a grueling biopsy to pull out as much tissue as possible to determine if Hodgkins disease was back. But Michael's only thought was the assembly at Pinetree Way elementary two days later.

The Grade 4 student wanted to play one of the songs he had written and say a few words to his school mates.

The audience of more than 500 students and adults in gym at Pinetree Way listened to him in silence.

"I'm sorry for the way I'm standing and talking," Michael said, "but I've just had surgery and it still hurts to keep my head up."

His message was simple. "To the healthy children – I know you're all good-hearted and feel badly for the others. You have to live a normal life, but don't think you're better than the sick children, those in wheelchairs. Don't treat them differently."

To the sick children he said: "Don't give up hope. Your mind is very powerful. Tell your body you'll make it. Be positive and keep faith. Remember, you've been through one tough time and when another one comes along, tell yourself, `I will make it again.' Work harder, think harder and pray harder."

Michael has poured his feelings into songs he has written and helped compose, and three have been recorded.

A compact disc, which is yet to be titled, is in the works, but *Make a Difference* the name of one song may be the title as this is Michael's goal: to make a difference.

Michael said he wants it to make "lots of money – but not for me. For the other kids." He plans to donate the proceeds to cancer research.

Until a year ago, Michael was one of "the healthy children." Then the headaches began, along with dizzy spells. He was more tired than usual. One day last summer, while he and friends were on a paddle-wheeler on Whonnock Lake, Michael fainted and fell into the water.

His friend Brodie Young, 9, pulled him to shore and helped revive him.

Parents Gloria and Domenic took their son in for a checkup and when the diagnosis came back, it wasn't good. Michael had Hodgkin's disease. This disease of the reticular and lymphatic tissues most

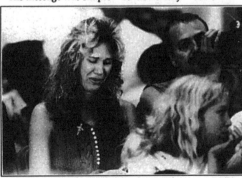

Michael Cuccione's mother wipes away a tear while an emotional father videotapes his speech

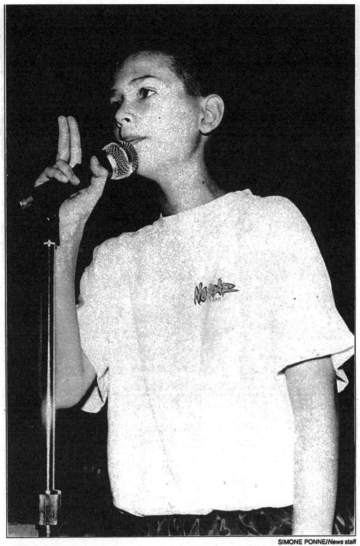

SIMONE PONNE/*News* staff

Michael Cuccione... "I'm going through it again, but this time I'm locking the door.

often affects young men.

"If there was a type of cancer to get, it would be this one," Michael says. "It's the most curable."

Michael is a aware of what he must now go through: constant medical exams, surgery, chemotherapy, possible hair loss as well as possible breakdowns in his immune system, but this awareness hasn't stopped him from going on with his life and doing something to benefit others.

This is how he feels about the cancer: "It's like my brother and sister wanting to come into my room. It's my room, so I keep them out. With my body, it's the same thing.

"I've overcome this the first time, and I will again. But the first time, I forgot to lock the door. I'm going through it again, but this time I'm locking the door."

Three weeks before the end of school a routine exam and bloodwork showed no trace of cancer. A chest x-ray, however, did; five or six spots showed around his lungs and heart.

Three days after speaking at the year-end assembly, Michael returned to Children's Hospital for surgery and chemotherapy. He is still there. His words come back like a prayer. "Tell your body you'll make it. Be positive and keep the faith."

disease and achieve his goals radiated from his eyes. "I'm going through it again, but this time I'm locking the door," he vowed. The school wished him well by giving him a long standing ovation.

Lock The Door *was to become his third song. The local newspaper wrote an article about this event and included two photos—one of Michael and another of Domenic and Gloria. My daughter is weeping. I have never seen such pain on her face. Every time I look at the photo, I cry myself.*

 June 30, 1995

Michael is scheduled for surgery tomorrow. He is to have his central line hook-up inserted into his chest wall. Dr. Anderson phoned Gloria and told her to bring Michael in tonight, as the operation will be performed early tomorrow morning. Michael was upset because Domenic, Gloria, and his Uncle Mike had planned on taking him to a BC Lions football game this evening. The problem was solved by taking Michael to the hospital after the game.

Michael was glad he attended the game. The Lions won over Baltimore 37-34. There was a raffle for an authentic Gordie Howe picture, complete with his statistics and his personal autograph. What a treasure! Domenic entered Sophia, Michael, and Steven's names in the draw. Steven won. Unselfishly, he let Michael put the picture up in his bedroom.

At midnight our six weeks of incredible stress began. Domenic couldn't concentrate on anything but helping his son through the hardest time of his life. He has to take a few months off work to be with Michael. We are very lucky because Domenic's employers are highly supportive and can see how devastated Domenic is feeling. It is not possible for him to work at this time. Michael has also made it clear that he will need the

full support of both his parents to get through what lies ahead for him.

Domenic and Gloria will stay with Michael as much as the doctors will allow. I will help keep up the home front.

Chapter 8

Here We Go Again

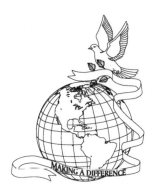

 July 1, 1995

Michael underwent his fourth operation in a week to install the central line. Unfortunately, it took two incisions before they could do the connection successfully. The way Michael has handled this past week is incredible to me.

 July 2, 1995

Michael was allowed to come home for an overnight stay. Physically, he looked like he had been through World War III. However, his good spirit was intact, for he was still smiling, singing, and cracking jokes.

 July 3 1995

Michael started his first chemotherapy session today. He was given seven grams of Cyclophosamide in four hours. The normal dose is one gram in a month. As a result of the chemotherapy, Michael was violently ill. Gloria was afraid that he would not be able to breathe due to his constant retching. She said his eyes kept rolling back. He has to be given fluids continually, to prevent dehydration and to prevent cystitis. It will be a miracle if he survives this.

Dr. Anderson said it is crucial that at least 80 percent of the cancer cells be destroyed to help ensure that the bone marrow transplant is a success. If signs of cancer are still present, Michael will need yet another dose of chemotherapy.

One of the possible side-effects of Cyclophosamide is cystitis. This is a condition in which the wall of the bladder starts breaking away, causing blood clots in the urine.

 July 4, 1995

Remarkably, Michael made an instant recovery from yesterday's chemotherapy treatments. He is doing fine , and is looking forward to going home tomorrow for 11 days. Michael has had the first G-CSF injection administered. They will need to be continued when he is at home, so Domenic was shown how to give the injection. The G-CSF is injected under the skin and into the fatty tissue. This will stimulate the bone marrow to push the granulocytes (stem cells) into the peripheral blood, where it will be possible to harvest Michael's cells. In turn, this will increase the white blood cell count and help curb infection, making it possible to maintain the intensive chemotherapy schedule.

 July 5, 1995

Michael was discharged from the hospital to go home. As soon as he arrived he went straight to the washroom. He had begun passing blood clots through his urine and he was experiencing a painful burning sensation. He called his mother and told her what was happening.

It appeared likely he would have to make an immediate return to the hospital. Michael asked if he could go up to his room, just for a few minutes, to feel what it was like to be in his own bed again.

While Michael was lying down, Gloria phoned the oncologist to tell him what was occurring. He said to bring Michael into the hospital right away, because he might have cystitis. If so, it would be necessary to administer fluids to flush the clots from Michael's bladder. Peridium would also be given to help relieve some of the pain. Gloria took Michael back to the hospital. Unfortunately, a diagnosis of cystitis was confirmed. Gloria stayed the night with Michael.

Once again, Domenic and Gloria began taking turns remaining overnight at the hospital.

 July 9, 1995

Domenic's sister Rena and her husband Vince are celebrating their 25th wedding anniversary. I have offered to spend the night with Michael at the hospital, in order that Domenic, Gloria, Sophia, and Steven can attend the party. I was glad to do this for I was eager to have Michael to myself.

We had a nice time. I picked up two movies and we spent from 3 p.m. until 11:30 p.m. playing games and watching movies. We were interrupted by Michael's frequent need to urinate. He was on the hydrating system because there were still blood clots in his urine. He will not be allowed to come home until this condition improves considerably.

On one occasion when Michael was going through this performance he stated firmly, "One day, when I get better— and I will get better—I will be telling my children about this." I prayed silently that he will be able to do just that.

 July 10, 1995

The chemotherapy has started to take effect, causing Michael's condition to deteriorate. He had a bad nosebleed this afternoon, which necessitated a blood transfusion. The chemotherapy has destroyed the clotting capabilities of his blood. Something more to worry about! Could Michael start off with Hodgkin's and end up with something else?

Even with all the testing that takes place with donated blood, there is still cause for concern. We know that it is impossible to screen out all potential problems. A severe blood shortage is expected next week. How is this shortage going to affect Michael when he needs blood transfusions?

 July 14, 1995

Michael had blood work, a CT Scan, and a pulmonary test done today. Although the pulmonary test showed a 20 percent loss in lung capacity, Dr. Anderson was generally pleased with the results. The CT Scan indicated that the cancer has practically disappeared. We are pleased that treatments will be proceeding to the next step. We can only hope that Michael's lungs will not get any worse.

 July 15, 1995

Michael was allowed to come home for five hours. He was craving a home cooked meal, so Gloria prepared a nice Italian dinner for the family.

Afterwards, I drove Michael back to the hospital and spent the night with him, to give Domenic and Gloria a break. We rented two movies on the way back to the hospital and we watched one of them that evening.

Michael was re-connected to the hydrating machine, which he has nicknamed "George". In order for Michael to go anywhere when he is in the hospital, he will have to unplug George from the wall and they will go together.

 July 16, 1995

In the morning, Michael watched the second movie while I read a book about bone marrow transplants. The information in it confirmed what Dr. Anderson has already told us. I read that Michael has a 20 to 50 percent chance of surviving this procedure. Even if he does survive, he could be limited physically. There is no guarantee that the Hodgkin's will not come back.

When I look at my wonderful grandson, I want to imprint on my memory every detail of him, in case the memory will be all I have left. Every time I think about the situation, my heart races, my throat closes off so I can barely swallow, and I can feel myself hyper-ventilating. I have never known such terror in my life!

After the movie, Michael and I played some games. He beat me at all of them. When the doctor said that he could go home for four hours, he was delighted. He asked for Italian sausages and prawns for his dinner. His friend Richie came over to be with Michael. They are such close friends and they had a great time together.

When Michael and his mother left at 6:30 p.m. to go back to the hospital, Michael cast a wistful look over his shoulder at all of us. He was, no doubt, wondering when he'll ever be back to stay.

 July 17, 1995

The harvesting of Michael's healthy stem cells began, all four hours of it. A pheresis machine, which Michael called "the washing machine," collected the healthy stem cells. Michael became quite involved in the process. He took on the job of cleaning the lines before they were hooked up to the machine. After the lines were connected, Michael's blood went through the machine. The new stem cells were retrieved and the rest of the blood was then returned to his body. He managed his usual smile while the procedure was being done. When the four hours were over, a bag of blood containing the life-saving stem cells were by his side.

That night he came home for a few hours, but it was no wonder that he looked very tired. For once he didn't mind going back to the hospital.

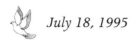 *July 18, 1995*

Michael spent one more day with the "washing machine."
After this was finished, he was finally allowed to come home
for a few days. Soon the most dangerous stage of his

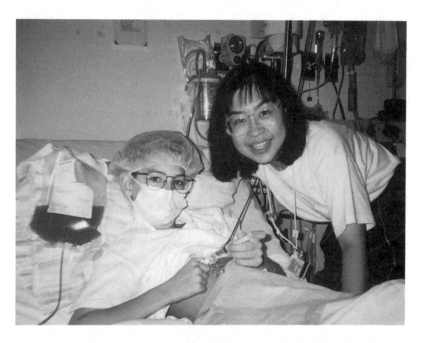

*A nurse watches Michael clean the line following
the procedure to harvest his life-saving stem cells.*

treatments will begin. We savour every moment that we have
with him now.

It is nearing July 25th, Steven's seventh birthday and the
anniversary of the first day we learned of Michael's cancer. I
decided to take Steven to see a roller-blade hockey game, the
Vancouver Voodoos vs. the Anaheim Bullfrogs. I knew that
Steven would enjoy it as he has been a whiz on roller blades
since he was three years old. He had a great time. There was a
barbecue and free roller-blade skating for an hour and a half
before the game started. The Voodoos won the game 11-5.

When we arrived home at 11 p.m., Michael was there. It was so good to see him!

 July 20, 1995

I did something special for Michael. He had been wanting a particular Super Nintendo game. I phoned around and finally found one. He was thrilled and he spent much of his remaining stay playing it with Steven. I was glad to do something to make him happy.

His hair has started to fall out again, just when it had returned to normal. Now he is back to square one.

 July 23, 1995

We have two more days to enjoy Michael being at home. Even with his hair falling out he looks so well, so normal. But he is facing so many risks, with land mines every step of the way. Will he ever come back to us again? If he does, will he be disabled in some way? Will this horrible disease come back? Michael must be wondering about these things, too, for he has started working on his fourth song, *I Don't Wanna Say Good-bye*. He is probably thinking about how his death would affect the rest of us and what it will do to his future plans. He is so determined to get the CD produced and begin making a difference!

There was a party to celebrate the birthdays of Steven and his Uncle Mike. We decided to celebrate early so Michael could be present. As usual, he circulated among the family members, joking and laughing. He wore his Grizzlies hat to cover his progressing baldness. Scars from his operations were visible above his T-shirt, yet Michael was totally unconcerned about it all. He enjoyed himself thoroughly.

 July 24, 1995

Steven had a birthday party with his friends at a novelty entertainment centre. Michael, Richie, and Sophia and her friend, Erin, came along. Michael is so pleased that he has been able to attend both of Steven's parties.

Later, Michael and his father returned to Children's Hospital. We had tried to get an overnight pass for Michael, but we were unsuccessful. Michael has to spend the night in the hospital to prepare for the ordeal that will begin tomorrow.

Chapter 9

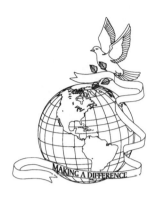

The Bone Marrow Transplant

 July 25, 1995

It is Steven's seventh birthday and Michael's first day of renewed chemotherapy to kill off his bone marrow. It is hard to believe that so much has happened to us in the last year. We ask for God's help to deal with this crisis. I believe that God answers our prayers by giving us the strength, on a daily basis, to get through all of the difficulties.

On July 31, following six days of chemotherapy, Michael will undergo the transplant procedure. Domenic and Gloria will alternate spending the next six nights with Michael until he is moved to Isolation for the Bone Marrow transplant.

In the meantime, there are the other two children to be concerned about. One good thing is that Sophia and Steven are very positive, and believe that Michael is going to make it. We also have great family support. Sophia will stay most of the summer with her aunts and uncles, and spend time with her cousins. Since Steven is primarily in my care, I will take him to roller-blade hockey games and swimming lessons to keep him occupied while his mother and father are at the hospital.

Today when we returned home from Steven's game, I decided to phone Children's Hospital to see how Michael was handling his chemotherapy. When my daughter picked up the phone, I could hear Michael's moans and crying in the background. This was the first time that Michael has shown this much discomfort. He was suffering a strong reaction to the chemotherapy. The severe itching was unbearable. My daughter had to hang up the phone and get him some help. About an hour later, she phoned back to tell me that Michael was sleeping. The medication given to him had relieved the pain and itching.

I have been warring with my conscience for some time over my plans for a ten-day trip to visit my brother and his family, in Belleville, Ontario. This trip was planned before learning of the return of Michael's cancer. Should I cancel my trip or will I be deserting my family when they need me? I wouldn't be very good company when I am so worried about Michael. I have second thoughts. I can see that my help is very much needed so I will postpone my trip.

 July 26 & 27, 1995

Michael's chemotherapy does not seem to be bothering him as much today. He is continuing to receive medications which are relieving the nausea and itching. Domenic and Gloria are looking very drained from this week's events. They have been missing Sophia and Steven and want to spend some time together, so I decided to help out by spending time at the hospital with Michael.

 July 30, 1995

Michael has completed his six days of chemotherapy. He has now been moved into an isolation room to prepare for the bone marrow transplant.

Everything will have to be completely sterile to avoid infection because Michael's immune system will be nonexistent. He will have no white blood cell count after the transplant. For this reason, no one will be allowed to stay with him overnight and the number of visitors will be limited. While Michael is in isolation, a physiotherapist will help him with exercises to strengthen his muscles. A nutritionist will work with Michael, attempting to provide him with appealing food.

Anyone entering the transplant room had to carefully observe the sterilization procedures. This included scrubbing their hands for two minutes with disinfectant soap, putting on a hospital gown and special slippers, and disinfecting with alcohol any items taken into the room. Even Michael's clothes brought from home had to be washed in extremely hot water. Food would be prepared in a special way so it would be safe to eat.

Many activities are available to help Michael occupy his time if he is well enough to do them. There is already a video and a Nintendo machine inside the isolation room. Michael will be able to enjoy movies, Nintendo games, board games, and cards. They have TV bingo for the patients and their visitors, with prizes for the winners. A recreational therapist will come in with arts and crafts for Michael to work on when he wants a change in his routine.

I spent the day at home catching up on odd jobs. Gloria came home and prepared Michael's clothes to be taken back to the hospital. As she took his clothes from the dryer, she fell to her knees, sobbing, wondering what was ahead for Michael.

Michael is facing many risks. No wonder we are all terrified that he might not make it through the coming weeks!

Michael says the "old" Michael is gone. The chemotherapy has seen to that. Tomorrow is the beginning of the "new" Michael. He is to be among the first at B.C.'s Children's Hospital to have this type of bone marrow transplant. It differs from an un-related donor transplant in that the transplant is an infusion of the patient's own stem cells, versus using the bone marrow of un-related donor. The 'newness' of this procedure also explains the extra cautionary procedures re sterilization.

 July 31, 1995

Today was a big day for Michael. The bone marrow transplant was this afternoon. Michael was 'rescued' with the previously harvested stem cells.

Just before the procedure, Michael asked his mother to play a song called *You Are Not Alone* during the transplant.

He received four vials of blood containing his stem cells through his central line. While the procedure was taking place, he experienced incredible pressure throughout his veins and in his head. He felt like he was going to explode.

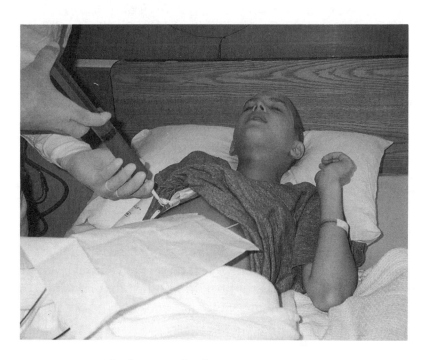

Michael receives his bone marrow transplant.
July 31, 1995

Unlike most people, Michael did not experience any vomiting during the procedure. He was mildly sick, just once, after the transplant. He managed this by exercising a great deal of self control. Music seems to soothes Michael's soul. His ability to concentrate on the music and relax was a great asset.

It will take time before the blood carrying Michael's stem cells finds its way to where the new bone marrow will reproduce.

There is a countdown after a bone marrow transplant. The days are numbered day 0, day+1, day+2, day+3, and so on. After three consecutive rises in white blood cell count, the patient is officially on "step-down" and is on the road to recovery.

One hundred days after step-down, barring any setbacks, the patient is considered to have recovered. Until then, there is the ever-present danger of infection, hemorrhaging, and organ failure.

 Aug. 2, 1995

<u>Day+2</u> Michael was told that tomorrow morning they will be inserting a tube through his nose down to his stomach. The rationale behind this is he might develop mouth and throat sores. If sores develop, they will make eating and swallowing so excruciating that morphine will be needed for pain control. To circumvent the issue of Michael not receiving adequate nourishment, they plan to insert the tube, even though no sores are present. Michael is determined that he will not get these mouth sores, and that he will be able to continue eating on his own. He doesn't see the need for this tube and is not looking forward to the procedure.

 Aug. 3, 1995

<u>Day+3</u> The tube connection was post-poned until this evening. It was inserted with no anesthetic. Michael found it

most uncomfortable. He was more or less in a daze for the next couple of hours. I was wondering what they were going to do to him next.

Michael told Gloria about two things that had happened. He described a vision that had been particularly vivid in his mind. In it, he was lying on his bed, with all his family surrounding him. He was trying to talk to them, but they could not hear him. He also made mention of another occasion when he had felt his body elevating from the bed.

When Michael told his mother about what he had been experiencing, she suggested that they pray about it. Michael's prayer went along these lines: "I know that it must be beautiful up there, God, but I am not ready to go yet. There's so much that I want to do. Please just get me through this as fast and as easily as possible."

He asked his mother if there was something that she would like to add. Choking back tears, trying to remain calm, Gloria said softly, "You've said it all, Michael." She saved her tears for the drive home, as she had done each night after leaving the hospital.

I have read that dreams like Michael's can occur to a person in the face of death.

 August 4, 1995

<u>Day+4</u> Michael received a visit from his Uncle Mike and Aunt Carla. It was highly emotional for all of them. His aunt and uncle painfully realized that it was too difficult at this time for Michael to have them visit. Michael was neither physically nor emotionally up to having them there. On top of everything else, the cystitis has returned with a vengeance.

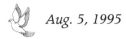 *Aug. 5, 1995*

<u>Day+5</u> I decided to spend it with Michael. I didn't know if I could handle the job or not, but that has never stopped me from tackling anything before. When I arrived at the hospital, Michael had just finished breakfast. Although he did have a good appetite, he was having difficulty eating because of the nasogastric (NG) feeding tube. Its presence was frustrating him terribly. He was quiet and withdrawn; I could see that he was feeling down. He was also experiencing severe diarrhea and stomach cramps.

Later, when he started to eat lunch, a few drops of blood began coming from his left nostril, the one without the NG tube. Since his blood had no clotting ability, I feared another one of his severe nosebleeds was starting. Luckily, the bleeding stopped, but itching set in. Medication was required and this helped him to get to sleep, but his rest was constantly interrupted as a result of the cystitis and diarrhea.

About 5:30 p.m., when Michael was attempting to eat his dinner, he became extremely faint. I rang the buzzer and a nurse rushed in and immediately started blood platelet transfusions. Shortly after that, Domenic and Gloria arrived. I realized that the best thing I could do was go home. Michael needed to be alone with his parents at this time. I looked at the machine that was recording his blood pressure. It showed his blood pressure as 98/54. I drove home in a daze. Were we going to lose him?

I phoned shortly after I arrived home. Thankfully, the blood platelets had stabilized him. I breathed a sigh of relief. The respite did not last long. Michael became incredibly nauseous. He vomited everything, including the NG tube reaching from his right nostril to his stomach. The nurse removed the part of the tube that remained as it was threatening to choke him. I am glad that I was not there for that part of the evening. I do believe that would have been the death of *me*.

Aug. 6, 1995

<u>Day+6</u> Michael continues to experience considerable discomfort, due to severe itching, diarrhea, stomach cramps, and blood clots in his urine. Within the past week he has been experiencing many sleepless nights. Tonight he felt the need to call home because he was lonely, scared, and homesick.

This was to be the only time Michael woke his parents during the night; still, Domenic and Gloria were glad they had told him to call at anytime.

 Aug. 8, 1995

<u>Day+8</u> For the first eight days, Michael's white blood cell count was nonexistent. He was receiving blood transfusions to increase his blood platelets. Something that is comforting Michael is that the NG tube has not been replaced. He is enjoying a good appetite. In fact, the nutritionists are surprised to see how much Michael has been able to eat following the transplant. The expected mouth and intestinal sores have not appeared. Frequent mouth wash treatments have helped Michael to prevent them.

 Aug. 9, 1995

<u>Day+9</u> Michael has had some wonderful news! There have been three consecutive rises in his white blood cell count; therefore, he is on official step-down. This means he can now leave his isolation room for short periods of time, though he is not yet strong enough to enjoy this privilege. Step-down also signifies that the transplant is working. One of Michael's nurses told him he has set a record of being the fastest patient on the ward to reach step-down. Many of the problems that he has been experiencing are diminishing, except for the blood clots in his urine.

Aug. 12, 1995

<u>Day+12</u> I stayed with Michael again. The cystitis was still troubling him. Due to the increased amount of fluids he was receiving, he was urinating every 20 to 30 minutes. Urine samples had to be tested to determine if the blood clots were increasing or decreasing. The doctor indicated to Michael that if not for the cystitis, Michael would be able to go home. This was very upsetting news for Michael because he would love to come home, and there was no way of knowing how long the cystitis would last.

On a brighter note, Michael left the isolation room for the first time. Gloria took him by wheelchair to a room where he enjoyed a nice soak in a tub. It relieved some of the tension he felt, and helped him to relax.

Sophia and Steven came for a visit. It was the first time they had seen Michael since his transplant. They felt bad for what Michael was going through, but they stayed optimistic that he would soon be home to stay.

 Aug. 13, 1995

<u>Day+13</u> Last night when Domenic and Gloria were saying good-night to Michael, he said, "I can't do this anymore, I can't stay alone at night. Can one of you stay with me?" Because Michael had faced his ordeals so bravely, never asking for any special treatment, they knew this request was very important to Michael and his recovery.

When they asked the nurse if one of them could stay with Michael, she was extremely firm in her denial. They argued back and forth, until the nurse agreed to let Domenic sit on a chair in the room for the night.

Today Gloria went to the head nurse and told her that she felt Michael should be able to have someone with him at night. He was on step-down, and would already have been able to come home, if it were not for the cystitis. She emphasized to the nurse how important having someone stay with him was to Michael. It could even affect his ability to recover. The nurse agreed with Gloria and had a cot brought into the room.

Since then this rule has changed. Now, children who are on step-down can have someone stay with them during the night.

 Aug 15, 1995

When Michael had been receiving his chemotherapy treatments the first time, he had met a 13-year-old girl named Melinda Rose Hathaway. Immediately, they became fast friends.

Melinda always put others before herself. When she was in the hospital, she spent her time visiting other cancer patients, trying to give them encouragement. Michael was attracted to her compassion, her ever-present smile, and her cheerful disposition.

On Valentine's Day, 1994, Melinda had been diagnosed with Askin's Tumour, a potentially fatal form of cancer which invades the soft tissue of the spinal column. Her cancer had since been reasonably under control. Now, in the midst of Michael's ordeal, Gloria heard the unbelievably sad news that Melinda's cancer had become extremely active again. Gloria did not have the heart to tell Michael about Melinda until a later date. Melinda knew that she was not expected to live long, though she always tried to live life to the fullest.

<u>Day+15</u> Michael had his spirits lifted today. Melinda, his dear friend, paid him a visit. They had been planning to go to Camp Good Times together, but Michael's relapse had made it impossible for him to attend. They had a great time looking at the pictures Melinda had taken at camp. She presented Michael with a poem and also a Get Well Award that she had made at camp for him.

When Melinda learned of the return of Michael's cancer and the treatments he had endured, she wrote a poem for him:

In The Promise Of Another Tomorrow

In your darkest hour, in your deepest despair
We will be friends forever and I'll be there.
Through your accomplishments and frustrations,
You will not be alone, you'll be in my heart,
Because we're friends forever, through thick and thin.
Even if we have to start all over again,
There is a war to be won and believe me it won't be fun
You have to be strong in order to overcome the wrong.
Through our anguish and our pain, through our joys and
*   sorrows*
All in the promise of another tomorrow, you can never give
*   up, keep on fighting!*

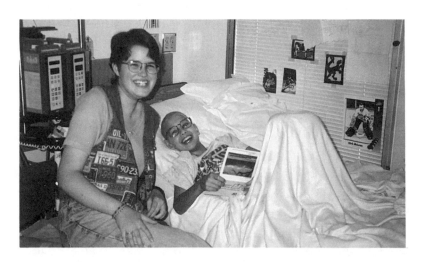

Michael's dear friend Melinda brings moral support
and laughter into the Isolation room.

Melinda's poem was very inspirational for Michael. Even though the reality of what he was going through was far more than he had anticipated, the moral support of those who cared for him was giving him the strength to endure his struggles.

 Aug. 17, 1995

<u>Day+17</u> There is light at the end of the tunnel for Michael. He has been granted a four-hour day pass. Gloria brought him home to see the rest of the family, who were eagerly waiting. Michael's tired eyes lit up as he came through the door. Our family was together again, even if only for a short time.

 Aug. 19, 1995

<u>Day+19</u> I went to the hospital yesterday morning and stayed with Michael until 4 p.m. today. I made sure that he ate well and that he did his mouth care. Michael seems to be one of the lucky ones—he still has not developed any mouth sores.

The cystitis was still bothering him and he was very tired. Having to urinate every hour and a half, around the clock, keeps him from getting enough sleep.

 Aug. 20, 1995

<u>Day+20</u> Michael was home for a six-hour pass this afternoon. He is still tired and weak but was glad to be home. Domenic went back with Michael and stayed the night with him.

 Aug. 21, 1995

<u>Day+21</u> Gloria brought Michael home for his first overnight stay in almost a month. Sophia had put a big

surprise in his bedroom for him. It was a huge bear, with "I Love You" stitched on a heart attached to the front of the bear. When Michael looked in his bedroom, he was touched by his sister's thoughtfulness.

Michael rested his frail body on his bed. He had lost ten pounds and is now down to 75 pounds. He was looking very weak and tired. The cystitis is nearly under control, but Michael still had to consume large quantities of fluid. This meant that he still has to get up twice during the night and drink a litre of water each time.

 Aug. 22, 1995

Day+22 Gloria made Michael an omelette for breakfast before going back to the hospital for further tests.

"What kind of cheese did you put in this omelette?" Michael inquired.

"Cheese slices," Gloria replied.

"I told you I only like brick cheese in my omelette," Michael said petulantly. "Have you forgotten already?"

My heart lurched. Are people so soon forgotten after they are gone? In time, would we forget the little things that went together to make up Michael, if we lost him? Was he expressing this fear by making that remark? I pray that we will never have to find out the answers to these questions.

Later, when Gloria got to the hospital, she was told that Michael would be able to come home very soon. Before he can do this, we have to clean the house from top to bottom, sterilizing everything, as Michael's immune system is suppressed. We are so glad that Michael's aunts are helping us with this job.

 Aug. 24, 1995

Day+24 This is a very big day for Michael and all of us! He is finally coming home to stay. Domenic and Gloria can now let go of the pain they felt every time they had to walk past

Michael's empty bedroom. What a great feeling for the whole family to be together again. The first few rounds of our fight have been won, but there are still a few rounds to go. You might say that we have won half the battle.

Chapter 10

Post Transplant

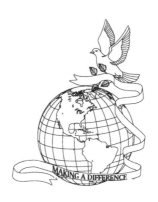

 Sept. 6, 1995

School has started without Michael. Instead, he returned to Children's Hospital for day surgery, to have his central line removed. While he was under the full effects of anesthetic, he

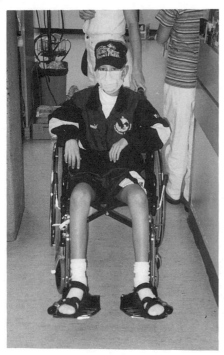

started coughing violently. Every muscle in his body was strained so badly that, combined with his frail condition, he was unable to walk. *He had to be carried up and down stairs for the next few days.*

He is very weak, so he is spending much of the time through the day sleeping. Due to the ever-present danger of infection, he requires home schooling with a tutor.

Five weeks post-transplant Michael is still very weak.

Sept. 8, 1995

I was finally able to take my trip to Belleville, Ontario. After the incredible stress of the previous two months, I am welcoming the ten days away.

 Sept. 18, 1995

I enjoyed visiting my brother and his family, with whom I have always been very close. I came back feeling renewed and I was looking forward to seeing the family.

I was shocked when I saw Michael. He is pitifully thin and is scarcely eating or drinking. He has dropped from his original weight of 85 pounds down to a mere 59 pounds. He looks downright anorexic.

Michael had his Gallium injection today. He will have to have extensive testing done on Gloria's birthday. We are all hoping that we will receive positive results.

Much later, we were to learn how close Michael came to not making it after the transplant. Before his cancer treatments, Michael had a pulmonary count of 129 points, 29 points above normal. After the transplant, he had a count of 29 points. Over a year later, when Michael was having his pulmonary test, the specialist told him about this.

"What would have happened if I hadn't had those extra 29 points?" Michael asked.

"You wouldn't be here," the specialist replied.

A coincidence or a miracle? I am convinced that it is the latter.

 Sept. 21, 1995

Michael was referred to the Make A Wish Foundation shortly after he relapsed. This foundation grants wishes to

patients who have life-threatening illnesses. Michael's wish is
to meet all the cast of *Baywatch,* a television show he watches
every afternoon, and they have granted his wish. This would
be the thrill of a lifetime. Even though Michael's wish has
been granted, it must be postponed for some time. He is not in
any shape to travel.

 Sept. 22, 1995

Michael returned home from having his Gallium scan, CT
Scan, electrocardiogram (ECG), pulmonary and blood tests.
These test results will give us the first indication of how
Michael is doing. We are all on pins and needles waiting for
the call with the results.

About five o'clock we received the results from
Dr. Anderson. It appears that the bone marrow transplant has
been a success. It is Gloria's birthday and I couldn't have
asked for a better gift for my daughter to receive. I decided to
take the family to a nearby restaurant to celebrate. It did us
all a world of good to get out of the house.

 Oct. 2, 1995

Domenic, Gloria, and Michael had to return to the hospital
for a meeting with Dr. Anderson. An important decision has
to be made regarding possible radiation treatments for
Michael.

Dr. Anderson had a consultation with a team of specialists.
They are all strongly recommending that Michael have the
radiation treatments to help ensure that the cancer will not
return. Although they are highly reluctant to have this done,
Domenic, Gloria, and Michael feel that they had no choice.
They cannot risk having the cancer return.

Michael is to receive twelve radiation treatments around
his neck and sternum. Half of his heart and lungs will be in
the field of radiation. This procedure is extremely dangerous,
due to the risk of heart and lung damage, or of producing a
secondary cancer.

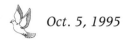 *Oct. 5, 1995*

Domenic, Gloria and Michael met with the radiologist. She explained the procedure. A cast of his body will be made to fit from the top of his head to his waist, in order to keep him from moving during treatments. These casts will be in two separate parts. One half will cover his back and the other half will cover his front. His body will be tattooed with small spots, front and back, to indicate where the radiation is to be directed. These tattoos will be permanent.

Domenic and Gloria were concerned about Michael's weight and his low pulmonary count. The radiation could cause side-effects such as nausea and more weight loss. Gloria wanted to wait until Michael became stronger before having these treatments done, but the specialist reminded her that if the cancer was going to come back, it would come back quickly. If these treatments are going to be effective, they have to be done right away.

Michael was able to take these treatments well, not dwelling on the consequences. We had been concerned about possible nausea affecting Michael's appetite, and causing further weight loss. Fortunately, he did not experience any problems with his appetite.

Shortly after Michael's chemotherapy, the bone marrow transplant, and the radiation treatments, he was given help which we feel is partly responsible for his recovery. Michael's friend Brodie and his family came to visit. Seeing how pathetically weak and thin Michael was, they realized the

seriousness of his condition. They recommended starting him on herbs from Enrich International.

Many testimonials regarding the dramatic improvement to the health of people suffering from various diseases can be found in this company's brochures. The principle involved is that when people like Michael cannot eat due to lack of appetite, toxicity or damage done to their digestive tracts, they can still swallow herbal pills or capsules. These pills provide nourishing food in its purest form. At the time, Michael was eating between 400 to 500 calories a day. With all the toxicity in Michael's body, the enzymes could not perform their digestive functions properly to nourish his body. His system needed to be cleansed completely of these toxins before he could get his appetite back and start gaining weight. The method of the herbal system of health care is to rid the body of toxins and provide the body with what it needs to restore and maintain its health. Michael was desperately in need of all these things.

The herbs Michael took (and is still taking) plus their benefits are outlined as follows:

Life Path   *Rids the body of toxins, helps tissue damage, increases the energy, appetite, and builds up the immune system.*

Chloroplasma   *High in beta-carotene, which builds up the body's immune system and increases body energy.*

C-Curity   *Rich in vitamin C. Activates cleansing enzymes in the colon and liver. Boosts the immune system.*

Native Legend Tea   *Soothes inflamed tissue and irritated membranes. Enhances digestion. It may assist in total internal body cleansing at the cellular level.*

Red Clover	*Purifies the blood. Rids the body of toxins and builds up the immune system. Some people believe it to be useful in fighting cancer, tumours, mucus build-up, multiple sclerosis, eczema, acne, and liver problems.*
White Oak	*Helpful in sore joints and weak connective tissues. It is believed to strengthen bones, muscles and connective tissue, and circulation.*
Acidophilus	*Helps increase the friendly bacteria in the colon, which are needed for the proper digestion of B vitamins. It can boost the immune system and reduce toxic waste in the large intestine.*

Within days of taking these herbs, Michael started getting his energy back and eating better. Soon he was gaining weight. A year later, he was back up to 85 pounds. We believe these products helped cleanse his body and fortify him against the toxins from the cancer treatments.

 Nov. 8, 1995

It is Michael's 100th day after his step-down. This is a big milestone and is a great cause for celebration! Michael had requested that we celebrate by having dinner at the restaurant at the top of Grouse Mountain. Symbolically, he has just climbed a huge mountain.

Earlier in the day, Gloria called the restaurant to check the visibility from the mountain top. She was told that it was not very good. By the time we arrived there that evening, the view was spectacular. The weather had become unusually clear and we hoped that this change forecast a bright future for Michael.

Thirty of his relatives came with us, as well as three special friends: Brodie, Richie, and Tyler. It was wonderful to see Michael joking and laughing at the table he shared with his friends.

 Nov. 10, 1995

Michael had a special celebration at home with his friends. They have all been so loyal to him throughout his illness. Michael's radiation treatments had just finished, so he had everyone sign the body casts used during treatments.

Michael reflected with Gloria on how much it had meant to him to have his friends come to the door after school to visit. During the long stretches of recovery time when he was confined at home, these visits were a highlight. They helped Michael to take his mind off his illness and to still feel part of his social group.

 Nov. 13, 1995

One of Michael's major goals had been to get well enough to be able to return to school. Michael announced to one and to all that tomorrow he is going back to school: "I know my body, and my body tells me that I am ready."

This announcement marked a monumental achievement and is an example of Michael's belief that if we set goals, it is possible to reach them.

 Nov. 14, 1995

Sure enough, instead of sleeping until noon, Michael got up, and by 8:30 a.m. he headed out the door, along with Sophia and Steven. Privately, we gave him until noon. No way. At noon he ate all the lunch that his mother took him and remarked dryly, "Thanks for asking me how my day is going." Michael was beaming from ear to ear. His mother could tell that he was enjoying himself. He came home with only four math questions for homework. He had been able to keep up with the rest of the class. What we had been dreading turned out to be a blessing.

 Nov. 17, 1995

Michael still has a way to go, however. This was made clear to him when he went swimming after school with Richie. Somehow, there was some jockeying for position in the line-up to get into the changing room and Michael was pushed to one side.

"Hey, take it easy," Michael firmly said.

"What's the matter, Ethiopian, can't you take a little shoving?" remarked one of the boys.

"As a matter of fact, I can't," replied Michael. "I've just had a bone marrow transplant."

"What's that?"

"It's a treatment for cancer. I've had the disease for a year and a half," replied Michael.

"Sorry."

Michael's parting comment was, "You shouldn't be calling *anyone* Ethiopian. Some people, like myself, can't help being thin."

I ached for Michael when he relayed the incident to me. I hoped the boys learned their lesson. That night, Michael told his mother and father what had happened.

"When am I going to be normal?" Michael cried, tears brimming in his eyes. "Everybody is dying all around me. Why does this world have to be so cruel?"

The bone marrow transplant has left Michael extremely thin. His back and leg muscles ache continuously. He cannot bend down to tie his shoes. It's not a surprise he is wondering if he will ever be normal again.

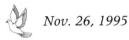 *Nov. 26, 1995*

Domenic, Gloria, and their children have just returned from a four-day trip to Whistler. The complimentary accommodations were provided by The Chateau Whistler Hotel through B.C.'s Children's Hospital. The family was given two connecting rooms with a view of the mountain.

They could ski from the hotel entrance to the ski lifts. Michael, although still thin and frail, surprised everyone by keeping up with them on the ski hills. When the family wasn't skiing, they spent their time sightseeing, shopping, going to restaurants, and swimming in the hotel pool. The fresh air and exercise did Michael a world of good, and it was great fun for the whole family.

Chapter 11

The Holidays

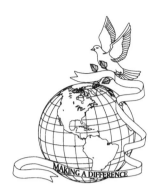

 Dec. 7, 1995

Michael is scheduled for a battery of tests including Gallium, pulmonary and ECG tests on December 15th. These tests will be recurring every three months, indefinitely, to see whether Michael is suffering from any ill effects due to his cancer treatments and to determine if he is still free of cancer. Each time, we will be holding our breaths, praying that the cancer has not returned.

Gloria has decided to postpone these tests until January 8, 1996, so Michael can enjoy his Christmas holiday and his birthday celebration.

 Dec. 17, 1995

Michael's school report card was outstanding. After all he has been through, and all the class time he has missed, he still brought home straight A's. This showed us the power of Michael's determination. We are extremely proud of him!

 Dec. 24, 1995

The family always takes turns having get-togethers. This year we spent Christmas Eve with Domenic's family. Everyone contributed a special dish to the Italian dinner. Michael was now eating a little better and particularly enjoyed the food.

Around midnight, many family members, including Michael, decided to go to midnight Mass. This was very fitting, since we were all so grateful to God for sparing Michael.

Following the church service, we left for home. Sophia, Michael, and Steven went to bed right away so that Santa could fill their stockings and leave their presents.

 Dec. 25, 1995

The next morning, about 10 a.m., Steven appeared at my bedroom door and announced that we were going to start opening presents. When we gathered together it looked like we were having a pajama party. As usual, everyone received many fabulous gifts.

At two in the afternoon, we all went to the home of Domenic's mother and father for another big Christmas dinner. Family and friends dropped by to visit. We enjoyed talking about the gifts that we had received. We played a few games and left for home around midnight. Everyone was getting quite tired from all the excitement except Michael, who was still going strong.

 Dec. 26, 1995

It might have been better if Michael had undergone his tests before Christmas, for try as we might, we cannot stop worrying about them. We would like to enjoy upcoming special occasions, but in the backs of our minds lurks the fear that Michael's cancer may possibly return.

 Dec. 27, 1995

Earlier in the fall, Domenic enrolled Steven in a hockey league. It is a sport at which Steven excels. With Michael feeling better, Domenic and Gloria have been attending Steven's hockey games. We could all see the positive impact this was having on Steven. Even his teacher commented on how much happier he seemed at school.

Today, Domenic, Gloria, Sophia, and Michael went to see Steven play in his hockey tournament. He had a great game and scored a few goals. Whenever Steven scored, the whole family proudly cheered from the stands.

Later on, Michael looked downcast. As happy as he was for Steven, perhaps he was comparing himself unfavourably to his eight-year-old brother. Steven is the picture of health and very active in sports—something Michael, no doubt, wonders if he will ever be again.

Trying to cheer him up, his mother started discussing plans for Michael's birthday party on January 5th.

"Maybe we can rent the Space Ball like we did for Sophia 's party," Gloria offered. Michael seemed pleased with this idea.

With the Space Ball booked, the birthday problem is solved.

 Dec. 31, 1995

Domenic and Gloria had to make a decision about what they wanted to do tonight to celebrate New Year's Eve. They had several invitations to go out, but Domenic's and Gloria's hearts were with their family. We decided to bring in the New Year with the children, so we went out to our favourite restaurant. After we came home from the restaurant, Domenic and the children went out to rent some movies.

While they were out, Gloria started to cry. She said, "What will happen if something shows up in his tests? I can't stop worrying about Michael's health. He's been through so much, and he can't take anymore. Nothing has seemed to have gone right for Michael. He deserves the best, but he has had so much bad luck."

I shared my daughter's anguish and tried to reassure her. Domenic and the boys returned. They were quite enthusiastic about the plans for the evening. Michael had a big grin on his face as usual. This helped to cheer Gloria up.

A friend of mine, Joanell, joined our family party about 10:30 p.m. We sang some songs, then as a special treat,

Michael sang *One Moment In Time*. After we danced to a few CDs, Michael was in pain so he lay down on the chesterfield.

Immediately, we surrounded him, fearing the worst, but he seemed to be breathing normally.

"Where is the pain?" Domenic asked. Michael reached down and started rubbing his abdomen. "You have a bit of indigestion due to all the food you ate tonight," Domenic said reassuringly.

About ten minutes later, Michael was up and brought in the New Year with the rest of us. There is a superstition that those who are with you on New Year's Eve will be with you throughout the coming year. We want all the insurance we can get that all our family will be together!

 Jan. 1, 1996

Today Gloria had Domenic's relatives over for dinner. It was a combination party for Domenic's and Michael's birthdays and New Year's Day.

The family members arrived around four in the afternoon. We enjoyed a large buffet dinner and spent the rest of the evening socializing with one another. At nine, the birthday cake for Domenic and Michael was brought out and everyone joined in singing "Happy Birthday". We are very thankful that Michael is with us to celebrate his 11th birthday!

 Jan. 4, 1996

This afternoon, Michael and Gloria were sitting side-by-side on the chesterfield. Michael was looking somewhat disappointed. His friend's mother had phoned and told Gloria that Michael's friend couldn't come over since their family was all recovering from the flu. The friend's mother meant well, and was right to fear subjecting Michael unnecessarily to the flu, but Michael was afraid many of his friends would avoid him for that same reason.

Jan. 5, 1996

Michael's birthday party turned out to be a great success. All of his plans went smoothly and the rest of the friends he had invited attended. This was very important to Michael because he doesn't want his illness to cost him any friends. He needs their support.

 Jan. 6, 1996

I've been sensing that Michael has some misgivings about being able to keep up with his peers physically. I thought I would give his ego a bit of a boost.

"I have never heard you sing *One Moment In Time* as well as you did New Year's Eve, Michael," I remarked. "Everyone was amazed."

Michael's face brightened. "I can still hold those notes, can't I?"

"You bet you can!" I said firmly.

Chapter 12

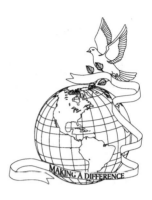

The Battle Continues

 Jan. 8, 1996

The day has come for Michael's tests; the emotions are high. Domenic, Gloria, and Michael left for Children's Hospital early this morning. Michael was having blood work, a CT Scan, and lung tests. He also received the injection to begin the Gallium test procedure. Michael's blood work is the best it has ever been. Everything was in the high normal range. His weight has increased, but the one cause for concern was that Michael's lung function was very low. Michael is suffering from residual lung damage which was causing inflammation in the lungs. The specialist felt that with the use of a Pulmicort inhaler this condition may improve.

While at the hospital, Michael wanted to visit his friend Stephanie. She is a 12-year-old girl who had received her bone marrow transplant just before Michael had received his. Stephanie's younger brother was a perfect match and had donated his bone marrow to her. Sadly, Stephanie has relapsed for the third time and is receiving chemotherapy. The treatments had robbed her of her hair once again. She was violently ill. She was curled up in her bed, frail and alone. Her mother and brother were on their way to the hospital from Prince George, British Columbia. Michael and Gloria did their best to comfort her. Seeing Stephanie so sick was difficult for them, especially since they were anxiously awaiting the results of Michael's tests.

They returned home to await Dr. Anderson's call giving them the important results of the CT Scan. When he phoned, we found out that he was unable to give us the results until tomorrow. Talk about nerve racking!

 Jan. 9, 1996

Michael went to school. It was agonizing for him to have to wait for the outcome of his tests. He told Gloria to phone the school right away when she knew the results.

At 1 p.m. the phone rang. It was Dr. Anderson. "Is it good news?" Gloria inquired breathlessly.

"The best!" Dr. Anderson replied. "Michael's CT scan is clear and his lungs show no spots whatsoever."

Gloria was ecstatic when she got the news. She burst into tears, but this time they were tears of joy.

The results eased our minds somewhat, although we will have to go to the hospital in two more days for the Gallium test.

Gloria phoned the school right away and asked to speak with Michael. When she told him the good news, he yelled, "Yes!" He returned to his class elated. Everyone joined in expressing their happiness for him.

 Jan.11, 1996

Gloria and Michael went back to Children's Hospital for Michael to have the Gallium scan. While they were waiting, they visited Stephanie again. Gloria and Michael brought her a jogging suit and a game. Stephanie was overjoyed. She and Michael played the game together and chatted like long-time buddies. It is amazing how easily Michael can interact with other cancer patients. But then he has a strong empathy for them.

 Jan. 12, 1996

Gloria and Michael made a special trip to the hospital to visit Stephanie again. She had used what little strength she had to go down to the gift shop to get Michael a gift. When she presented him with a car model, Michael was really touched.

"You're so nice, Michael. I thought all boys were mean until I met you. The boys I know are always teasing me and making fun of me," Stephanie said softly.

"I can't understand how anyone could be mean to you," Michael said.

That night, Domenic told Gloria of his concern for Michael to be seeing Stephanie when she was so ill. He was afraid it might be too hard on Michael at this time. Gloria reminded Domenic of how important Richie's loyalty was to Michael throughout Michael's illness. Richie himself had been afraid of becoming too involved with Michael, for fear that if Michael passed away, he would have a hard time getting over it. Richie's mother told him not to think about that, and just to enjoy being with Michael while he was here. After that, their friendship became stronger. Indeed, the whole school, especially the principal, has stood by Michael throughout his ordeal.

We got the good news. The Gallium test supported the CT Scan results. Indeed, Michael has been cancer-free for six months! This is the first big milestone since the transplant. The news eased our minds, for we remembered being told that if Hodgkin's was going to come back, it would come back very quickly.

Michael's follow-up appointments are scheduled to take place on a monthly basis.

 Feb. 4, 1996

Michael visited Stephanie again today. She gave him great news. Her leukemia is back in remission. She gets to return home to Prince George with her family. The sad part of all this is Stephanie's mother told Gloria that even though Stephanie is in remission, the doctors feel it is only temporary. They are fairly certain that she has only a few months to live. We can only keep hoping and praying for another miracle.

Gloria kept this part of the news from Michael. I'm glad that Michael and our family have been able to give Stephanie some happiness. She is such a live wire—a fighter all the way.

 Feb. 16, 1996

We are very upset. Michael had a bad asthma attack and felt faint. He still has a very low pulmonary count. It is difficult to say how much his lungs will recover. He attempted a basketball game and a gym class, back to back. Michael feels that he has to prove to himself, and others, that he can do everything he did before his illness. Domenic and Gloria told him not to be afraid to back off when he is feeling weak and tired. He has to give his system time to strengthen itself.

 Feb. 19, 1996

We had another scare about Michael. The school phoned about one o'clock to let us know that Michael had a very bad nosebleed. We were extremely concerned and went immediately to the school. Everything was under control, and we did notice that his blood clotted quite well. Let's hope that we have nothing more to worry about.

 Feb. 21, 1996

Michael fell at school and bruised himself so badly that he went into shock. Gloria was called to the school. Michael told her that he couldn't remember if he had tripped or if he had fallen down. Gloria went with Michael in the ambulance to Children's Hospital. After a thorough check-up it was determined that Michael was fine. We can't help but feel alarmed every time something happens to Michael.

Feb. 22,1996

Michael received some good news. He was chosen to be the BCTV/Dairy Queen Saturday's Child for the month of February. This monthly award is given to a child under eighteen who is deemed to be a positive role model for other children and who wants to make a meaningful contribution to society. Some of the qualities the award committee looks for include enthusiasm, ingenuity, kindness, commitment, resourcefulness, and a positive outlook. Michael certainly qualifies in all respects!

 Feb. 26, 1996

In preparation for the presentation of the Saturday's Child Award, Michael was video-taped at school with his friends, at a voice lesson, singing one of his songs, and in the recording studio. A touching part of the video was when one of Michael's close friends, Tyler, was asked about Michael. He promptly replied, "He's going to be the cure for this disease. He's the best kid I have ever known."

 Mar. 2, 1996

At 7 a.m. and 10 a.m., Michael was shown on BCTV broadcasts covering Michael's story and being presented with the award by Wayne Cox. Dairy Queen gave Michael a recognition plaque and a $1,000 gift certificate. Michael was asked what he was going to do with the money. Michael said, "As much as I could use a new pair of jeans, I am going to put this money towards my fund for cancer research." Michael was so natural and sincere that the TV hostess was moved to tears! The program was repeated on both evening news programs.

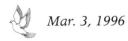 *Mar. 3, 1996*

Michael and his class went on a skiing trip to Whistler for the day. About 6:30 p.m., when Gloria went to school to pick Michael up from the bus, there was no one in sight. Thinking that the bus was late, she went back at 7:30. There was still no sign of a bus and school children. When she arrived home, she phoned the vice-principal to see what had happened. The news was not good. A blizzard had struck and the bus was stranded waiting for stuck cars to be cleared. Luckily, they were near a small town so the children were able to get something to eat and go to the washroom. It was 11:00 p.m. before the class arrived home. Meanwhile, all we could do was wait and hope they all returned home safely. It was one more episode in the ups and downs of Michael's life.

 Mar. 7, 1996

Michael went to Children's Hospital for another chest x-ray and pulmonary test. Again we prayed that everything is well with Michael. Thankfully, it is. While at the hospital, Gloria and Michael met Stephanie and her mother and brought them home to have dinner with us. Stephanie has been at the hospital, having some checkups. She looked well, but in the backs of our minds are the specialists' dire predictions. Still, we hope for a miracle for Stephanie.

 Mar. 8, 1996

Michael was invited by Enrich International to speak to five hundred distributors. Michael shared his story with the guests about how much Enrich products had helped him to recover and maintain his health.

Barry Borthistle, President of Enrich International, Canada, was in the audience. He was impressed both with Michael's ability to express himself and also by his powerful story. He invited Michael and his parents to attend the Enrich Convention taking place on a Caribbean cruise in January,

1997. Barry said to Michael, "You will be able to share your story with people from all over the world." What an honour!

Later, Michael turned the television on to watch the CTV news. He saw Melinda's parents being interviewed. Her father was describing Melinda's web site and the remarkable response it was receiving. Melinda's doctor spoke of her deteriorating health, but commented on how positive she was keeping every day. Her mother, Joanne, mentioned Melinda's nightmares about dying. Unfortunately, in Melinda's case, the nightmare is becoming a reality.

 March 30, 1996

Domenic and Gloria and the children returned from a two-week vacation to Florida. During the vacation, Michael was constantly coughing and had a fever. Domenic and Gloria were very concerned. They had hoped the warm weather would help Michael's condition. They still managed to have a great time, Michael being such a trooper.

The family stopped over in Toronto to visit some of Domenic's relatives, who were so happy to see them. They love Michael. They can't believe that the family has been through so much.

Michael has been anxious and easily irritated since coming back from the trip. We thought that he might be experiencing a let-down from his trip. In the evening, more light was shed on the reason for his moods.

"You didn't seem to be too happy when I dropped your lunch off today. Was something bothering you?" my daughter asked.

"Lots of things were bothering me today," Michael replied. "I feel so badly about Melinda and Stephanie."

No doubt, the awareness that both Melinda's and Stephanie's cancers are progressing made him worried about losing his friends.

Chapter 13

I Don't Want To Say Good-Bye

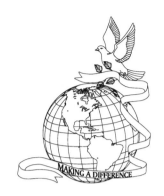

 Apr. 18, 1996

It has been nine months since Michael's bone marrow transplant and he remains in remission. He still looks slim, but his strength and energy levels are increasing.

Michael and his family were invited to the B.C.'s Children's Hospital Kick Off Party at the Granville Arts Theatre. This was a celebration to thank all of the major sponsors and supporters of the Children's Miracle Network Telethon. It was an honour for Michael and his family to be invited. Michael gave a speech to update everyone on his recovery from cancer and his future plans to raise money with his CD.

He thanked everyone for supporting the Children's Hospital Telethon, and sang *Make a Difference*. He received a long standing ovation. Dr. Leblanc, the surgeon who had done the biopsies during Michael's relapse, was in the audience. He hadn't seen Michael since he had performed the surgeries. He was amazed to see Michael looking so well, and couldn't believe that he was producing songs and expressing himself so eloquently. He asked Michael to speak and sing at a golf tournament fundraiser. Michael was only too happy to agree.

He was also invited to perform for the telethons on the multicultural network and UTV (Global Television). He'll be singing two of his songs at each of the performances.

Apr. 23, 1996

Gloria took Michael for his check-up at the hospital. Following the CT Scan, the specialist called Dr. Anderson for an immediate consultation. Gloria met with the doctor while Michael was having his chest x-ray taken.

The CT Scan had revealed a spot about one centimeter long at the bottom of Michael's right lung. Dr. Anderson saw that Gloria was extremely anxious. He tried to explain to her what the spot could be indicating. He asked if Michael had recently had a bad cough, or had been feeling otherwise unwell. Gloria remembered that Michael had been coughing a lot when they were in Florida. Dr. Anderson told Gloria that the specialist suspects that Michael might be fighting off pneumonia. It will not be until tomorrow that the specialists, after a conference, will be able to give a more definitive diagnosis. On the trip home, Gloria did her best to hide her fears from Michael.

We have not shared our concerns with him, but we think he knows something is wrong from the serious looks on our faces. Domenic feels bad that Gloria had received frightening news alone.

 Apr. 24, 1996

Gloria told me that she had stayed awake all night. Domenic tried to comfort her, but she cried intermittently throughout the night.

We received the word this afternoon. The specialists said that Michael still had a small spot on his lung. Nevertheless, they didn't feel that any further treatment was needed. The spot would likely clear up on its own.

Gloria decided to start Michael on a special herb that is supposed to clear any mucous that is lining the walls of his lungs. We were relieved by the news from Dr. Anderson and yet still afraid that it could be something else.

May 15, 1996

Domenic, Gloria, and Michael attended the golf tournament in support of Children's Hospital. Michael gave a speech praising the doctors and nurses at Children's Hospital and telling everyone about his continued work on his CD. Dr. Art Hister introduced Michael as a "natural talent." Michael sang one of his newest songs, *Lock The Door*.

 May 23, 1996

Michael went to Children's Hospital for blood work, pulmonary tests, and a chest x-ray. The blood work was great. We had been told that the blood platelet level might not return to the normal range after Michael's bone marrow transplant, but in fact the platelets are in the high-normal range. Also, the white blood cell count is in the high-normal range. His tests confirmed that he has successfully battled pneumonia during the last two months. His chest x-ray is clear. This shows that Michael's immune system is strengthening. What a great relief this is!

 June 1, 1996

Michael performed for the B.C.'s Children's Hospital Telethon on UTV today. He sang one of his songs. He also donated the $1,000 he had received as a recipient of The BCTV/Dairy Queen Saturday's Child Award.

 June 25, 1996

Michael had another CT Scan today. His test showed that he is completely clear of Hodgkin's Disease. Michael is ecstatic. He feels as if he has been given a new lease on life! Now he can really look forward to all the plans he has been talking about for the summer.

As Domenic, Gloria, and Michael were leaving the hospital, they saw Melinda and her parents in the parking lot. It was hard for them to see how much Melinda's health had deteriorated. Michael is wondering if Melinda will be able to come to Camp Good Times with him.

 July 8, 1996

Michael was happy today when he got a call-back for a commercial. We were surprised when Michael had said he wanted to start going to auditions again. I feel this is another one of Michael's personal goals. It's too bad he won't be able to attend the call-back, because he will be at camp.

 July 13 – 20, 1996

Michael is excited to be on his way to Camp Good Times at Sechelt, British Columbia. This is a camp for young cancer patients, children in remission, and their siblings. The children enjoy themselves thoroughly despite their afflictions.

Michael missed going to camp with Melinda last year because of his relapse. He was so happy to see Melinda at camp—morphine, wheelchair, and all. What a wonderful girl!

At one of the daily campfires, the children asked Michael to sing a song. He was more than willing. Before he sang, he dedicated his song, *Never Give Up*, to Melinda. Most of the children, including Michael, broke into tears.

Even though some of the children, like Melinda, are still suffering and terminally ill with cancer, they are able to put their agony aside while they enjoy normal childhood activities. This is what makes this camp so wonderful. It was nice for Michael to be temporarily problem-free, and to enjoy being with his friends for a few days.

 July 20, 1996

Michael came home from camp today. He had been reluctant to leave camp because he had felt so free there.

Michael raved about how awesome all the camp counsellors were, and said that this was something he would like to do in the future. He remarked on all the fun the children had playing practical jokes on one another.

 July 21, 1996

Stephanie's mother phoned to say that Stephanie has only a few days at the most to live. Gloria went to the hospital to try to comfort the family. Michael said he couldn't bear to see Stephanie suffering. He prayed for Stephanie that she would find peace.

Stephanie's mother wanted Gloria to help her phone some out-of-town relatives so that Stephanie could speak to them. Using what little strength she had left, Stephanie managed to say good-bye to each of her relatives.

 July 22, 1996

Stephanie passed away last night while snuggled up next to her mother. As far as our family is concerned, there can't be any greater hurt than losing a child.

 July 23, 1996

There was a small service for Stephanie. Michael's song, *When You Are Away*, was played, and he was given the privilege of saying a few words about Stephanie. Michael has lost another great friend—one more reason for him to continue his goal of helping to find a cure for cancer.

 July 24, 1996

Michael had blood tests and a chest x-ray. Tomorrow is Steven's birthday and the second anniversary of Michael's diagnosis of cancer.

Michael's tests and x-ray show he is still cancer-free. This is wonderful news which relieves our anxiety somewhat. We know that the longer the Hodgkin's stays away, the more hope there is of it not returning.

 Aug. 1 – 3, 1996

Michael is the introductory performer for Natasha Jaye, a very talented vocalist who is appearing at the Gastown Theatre in Vancouver. She has a degree in radio and television from Ryerson University. Her diverse singing styles have taken her from leading a house band in a Toronto pub to performing a lead role in a Gilbert and Sullivan stage production. It is a privilege for Michael to open her show by singing two of his songs.

 Aug. 10, 1996

We had a big party at our home to celebrate Michael being cancer-free for a year. It was a beautiful day, so all our guests, including our relatives and friends, Dr. Anderson and his wife, plus one of Michael's favourite nurses, enjoyed a big outdoor picnic. Michael gave a speech thanking Dr. Anderson and the staff at B.C.'s Children's Hospital for their excellent care, and saying how happy he was to have made it to his one-year milestone. Everyone became misty-eyed, including Dr. Anderson. He, more than anyone, realized what a miracle it was that we were able to have such a party.

 Aug. 13 – 23, 1996

Michael flew on his own for a ten-day trip to New York City to stay with Domenic's relatives. While there, he toured St. Mary's Children's Hospital, encouraging the young patients and spreading his message of hope. He told the patients, "Keep strong. Look ahead for the payoff. You just have to fight . . . and if the doctors give you any hope, fly with it."

Michael did a lot of sightseeing with his relatives. Two highlights were the Empire State Building and Times Square.

Gloria worried about Michael getting homesick. Personally, I worried more about how Gloria was handling Michael's absence. He couldn't have been too homesick. He gained three pounds while he was away.

The one detraction from Michael's enjoyment of his trip was Melinda's imminent death. With his parents, Michael had visited her before he left. She was at Canuck Place, a hospice for terminally ill children and their relatives. Melinda was almost totally paralyzed. The cancer had damaged her spinal column badly, yet she clung to life, wanting to be with her loved ones as long as possible. Although experiencing tremendous pain, she exemplified the poem she wrote for Michael: "You can never give up, keep on fighting." She has fought so valiantly!

 Aug. 25, 1996

Michael reached another milestone on the road to recovery. He performed at the Pacific National Exhibition (PNE) Talent Search Competition. This was Michael's first performance at a competition since he had his bone marrow transplant. His showmanship was spectacular. We were very pleased that he was one of the 12 finalists.

 Sept. 1, 1996

The 12 finalists performed at the PNE. Although Michael didn't place, the experience was highly beneficial and he did well, as there were originally 100 contestants. I was afraid that Michael might lose confidence as a result of not being one of the top three performers. He hasn't been working on his CD or practising his voice training exercises. He has been more interested in socializing with his peer group. He's not to be blamed for that—the last two years have kept him away from them much of the time. However, I felt that there was a lesson to be learned from this experience.

I mentioned that the winners of the contest had put in gruelling hours of practice to achieve their success. "How badly do you want to produce your CD, Michael?" I inquired, not too subtly.

"How badly do you want the book published?" Michael countered.

Michael and I had decided to write this book by this time. We had both been keeping journals. Michael provided me with details of the times when I was not present, especially when he was doing so much travelling and public speaking.

I realized that our goals were not going to be reached without some effort on both our parts. Michael started working on his fifth song, Never Give Up, *and I signed up for three computer courses. So far, I had been typing out this story on a manual typewriter. Michael and I share the belief that if you set your goals, you can indeed reach them.*

 Sept. 3, 1996

School started. Michael is cancer-free and looking great, with his dark curly hair and his big smile. (Before chemotherapy, his hair had been blonde and straight.) To put the icing on the cake, he is in grade six with two of his best friends, and he has a great teacher.

This afternoon, Michael was on Radio AM 104 for half an hour, telling his story, spreading his message, and talking about what the use of herbs had done for him. People kept calling in, wanting to get more information. Michael was very spontaneous in his answers. It was obvious that he wanted to be as helpful to the listeners as possible by supplying them with the information they were seeking. He has the potential to become a strong motivational speaker.

Sept. 10, 1996

Michael has gone back to karate after a two-year absence. It is wonderful to see him able to do this again. He can still handle the drills and moves well. This exercise will be very beneficial for the strengthening that his bones and muscles need.

 Sept. 15, 1996

We received the heart-wrenching news today that Melinda passed away. She suffered terribly, even with the morphine. Her heart finally stopped and released her from her pain.

Michael broke down in tears as the feelings of loss for another friend washed over him.

Melinda was so special that we want to give our readers a glimpse of what she was really like. This is why we have dedicated the next chapter to her. Her life has been truly an inspiration to all of us.

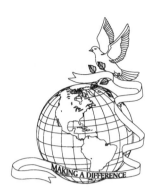

Chapter 14

Melinda Rose Hathaway
(May 19, 1981 – September 15, 1996)

On February 14, 1994, Melinda Rose Hathaway was diagnosed with Askin's Tumour, a rare and lethal form of soft tissue cancer that had invaded the structure of her spinal column. She was 12 years old.

Her condition was considered to be terminal. She was given only a few weeks to live. However, a punishing series of intense chemotherapy and radiation treatments, together with her own very strong will to survive, allowed her to continue on with her life for almost two and a half years after her diagnosis.

Melinda made the most of her last few months of life. Among other things, Melinda set up her home page on the Internet. Her father, David, supplied the technical computer knowledge, and her mother, Joanne, proofread and typed when Melinda was too tired. The first version was released on Valentine's Day 1996, the second anniversary of her diagnosis of cancer. The purpose of the home page was to provide "Cancer Kids" and their caregivers throughout the world with hope and any information that they might be seeking. Typically, instead of absorbing herself with her own problems, Melinda concerned herself with helping others.

When she started her home page, she hoped to one day reach a total of 500 visitors. At the time of her death, just seven months later, the count was 25,000 and growing, and by the end of 1997, it had reached almost 60,000—and is still growing.

Melinda loved to write. During her final two weeks, she and her father worked together on one final poem, which they completed on September 15, 1997, at 7:56 p.m., just one hour before she died. It is heart-wrenching. The poem is entitled "Wired." With all the morphine she had to take, she felt it was the one word that best described her condition.

Wired

I am a wounded child
Temporarily trapped
In the technology
Of modern medicine
But even though my eyes
May be clouded
They can still see
Far beyond the horizon
And with my ringing ears
I can hear sounds
That nobody else
Knows are there
My breath may come slowly
Forced into me through a mask
But the air is clean
And so very cool
And with someone else
Holding the pen
I can still write poems
And hope that they finish
Before the end.

More of Melinda's words, her poetry, and her true love and caring for seriously ill children can be found on her home page on the Internet. Her website has ensured that she will always be with us through the messages she has left behind. Michael is honored that his website is linked to Melinda's home page.

Melinda planned her whole memorial service, which was held September 23, 1996, at 3:30 p.m. in St. Catherine's Anglican Church in North Vancouver, BC. For songs, she chose *No Tears In Heaven* by Eric Clapton, *Because You Loved Me* by Celine Dion, and *One Sweet Day* by Mariah Carey. For a hymn, she chose *All Things Bright And Beautiful*. She gave Michael the honour of speaking at her service.

At the front of the church, there was a wonderful picture of Melinda. Michael said that all he could see was an angel. As he spoke about his friendship with Melinda, he held back the tears in order to be strong, but following the service, tears streamed freely down his face.

Hundreds attended Melinda's memorial service, while others from Australia, Sweden, Malaysia, South America, New Jersey, Texas, California, Ontario, Manitoba, and many other places that the Internet reached, sent messages of inspiration and love directly to her home page. Nearly all the messages were addressed to her as if she were still living. In that sense, through the magic of the Internet, she is still with us.

The words that Melinda included in her Order of Service are profound: ***"Cherishing a complete life does not necessarily require a complete lifetime."***

Chapter 15

The CD Is Released And The Foundation Is Established

After Melinda's memorial service, Michael's goals in life began to be realized beyond his wildest dreams. He finished his last song, Never Give Up, *which completed the songs required for his CD.*

Domenic and Gloria supported Michael fully in his goals of producing a CD. They put up $10,000 of their own money to have the CD produced. Several corporations graciously offered their support to market Michael's CD, Make a Difference. *Michael and his parents were very appreciative of receiving full support from Burger King across Canada, and Shoppers Drug Mart and Save-On-Foods in their BC locations.*

Photographs of Michael which appeared on the CD were done by Tonino Guzzo Photography. They were taken in Gastown in Vancouver, BC down a lane paved with cobblestones and near an iron doorway, symbolizing Michael's strength in dealing with his illness and 'locking the door'. More pictures and the words to his songs were included in a booklet inside the CD. Michael dedicated his CD to Melinda Rose Hathaway and "to all the kids at British Columbia's Children's Hospital, especially 3B ward."

 Oct. 5 – 12, 1996

Michael and the family spent a week in California for the fulfillment of Michael's wish through the Make A Wish Foundation.

Michael received a wish far beyond his expectations. The family met Jay Leno, and Sophia sat in one of the front seats in the audience during the show.

The greatest event of all was being allowed on the set of *Baywatch*. David Hasselhoff and the cast of *Baywatch* were wonderful to the whole family. Watching the video of this, you would have thought the Cuccione family members were the celebrities!

They sat Michael in a director's chair in the middle of all the action so he could watch the filming of the episode. David and all the cast members were signing *Baywatch* cast pictures, posters and magazines for each of the children. The make-up artist painted tattoos on Michael and Steven. Michael was allowed an appearance on the episode they were shooting.

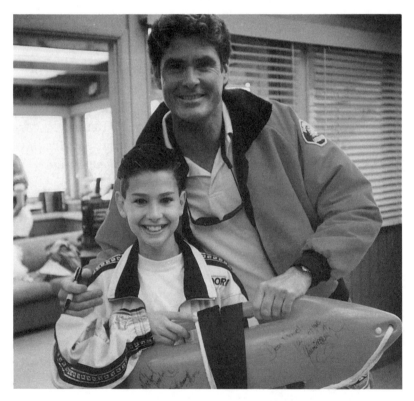

Michael's Baywatch *wish is granted:*
David Hasselhoff presenting Michael with an autographed rescue cannon.

There was a cart full of complimentary delicious treats. The cast included the family in the breakfast and luncheon times. David allowed the family full access to his trailer for the day if they wanted it.

David took time out to get to know Michael. He told Michael that when he was travelling on business, he would go to visit children in hospitals around the world to try to help them forget their problems for a while. He told Michael about Charlie Hays, a boy with terminal cancer who had spent a lot of time on the set of *Baywatch*. David said that he had been really touched by Charlie's story.

David gave Michael a signed copy of his own CD and Michael took this opportunity to tell David about the CD that he was going to produce. David requested a copy of the CD when it was ready. Fortunately, the family had brought a demo tape of Michael's songs and a package of news articles telling about what Michael had been through in the past two years. Gloria gave these to David.

Gloria was very surprised when a call to their room from David Hasselhoff came through the next morning. Apparently, his daughter had been playing Michael's demo tape most of the previous night and had enjoyed it very much. This must have given David an idea. He told Gloria that he was going to try to include Michael in one of the episodes of *Baywatch,* singing one of his songs — probably *Make a Difference.* As David put it, nothing was carved in stone, but if anyone could swing it, he could. This would benefit Michael's cause a great deal, as it would help create an international awareness of the need to support cancer research.

 Oct. 23, 1996

Michael and his family have returned from their California vacation. Michael is back performing. Today he sang at the Make A Wish Benefit. Michael expressed his gratitude to the Make A Wish Foundation for granting his wish to be on the set of *Baywatch.* He told the audience how wonderful it is to have a favourite dream granted when one has a life-threatening illness. He was especially grateful that his whole family had been included in the fulfillment of his wish. He spoke of his hopes and dreams to help find a cure for cancer, and of how he was going to use his CD as a vehicle for obtaining public support for his cause.

 Oct. 27,1996

A friend had asked Michael if he would mind speaking with another cancer patient to give him some information and support. Michael received a phone call from Alex, who at 24 was facing a bone marrow transplant. Alex's case was more complicated because he would be receiving a donor's bone marrow.

The bone marrow is harvested from the pelvic bone of the donor. The marrow is harvested by technicians who aspirate the marrow through bone marrow needles, which are repeatedly inserted into the pelvic bone. From then on, the procedure is the same as Michael's.

The risks would be greater for Alex, because in addition to all the dangers Michael had faced, there was also the danger of Alex's body rejecting the donated bone marrow. Alex had a very positive outlook, but I am sure that he found it comforting to talk to someone who understood. He and Michael related well to each other and became fast friends.

 Nov. 5, 1996

Michael and his family are thrilled beyond belief. They have held Michael's CD in their hands for the first time! One of Michael's goals is in his grasp, so to speak. There have been times along the way when everyone has wondered if this would only be a dream. Now that the dream is a reality, it is, indeed, cause for celebration. Sophia is so proud of Michael's CD that she took it and a portable CD player to school, so she could listen to it through the day and share it with her friends.

 Nov. 7, 1996

The first order for the CDs has been placed! Gloria has booked the Italian Cultural Centre in Vancouver for a CD Release Party on November 21. After their fantastic California holiday, the family is now getting down to business. Tickets are being printed, food ordered, a band hired. In preparation for the launch, Shoppers Drug Mart has generously hired a promoter who organized a CD signing with media coverage at one of their outlets. Michael has also appeared on BCTV, profile articles about him have appeared in the local papers, and local radio stations have played his songs and interviewed him. This all helped Michael to launch his CD.

 Nov. 22, 1996

The CD Release Party was a sold-out event, with 658 people in attendance. As guests were entering they were greeted by Michael, who was seated at a table autographing his CDs. While he was signing them, a man inquired about the price. Then the man presented Michael with a cheque for $1,000 payable to the Michael Cuccione Foundation. He asked Michael if that would cover the cost of a CD. Michael's eyes practically popped out of his head as he handed the man a CD and a cassette!

Wayne Cox, the BCTV broadcaster who had conducted Michael's Saturday's Child Award interview, had agreed to be master of ceremonies for Michael's special evening. Everyone commented on the fabulous job Wayne did.

The Canucks, Grizzlies, BC Lions, and Canadian National Soccer organizations donated prizes, including signed jerseys.

These items were auctioned off by Wayne Cox, with Michael hamming it up by modelling the jerseys and bouncing sports balls around the stage.

Michael was surprised and delighted when Alex and his family arrived at the party. Later in the evening, Alex bid on the Canadian National Soccer jersey, purchasing it for $850. It was very touching to find out that Alex was going to wear it for good luck during his bone marrow transplant. When Alex learned that Steven loved the jersey, he told him at the end of the night that he wanted Steven to have it after the transplant.

Dr. Anderson, Mike Cuccione, Sr., Domenic, Michael, and Barry Borthistle were featured speakers.

In Dr. Anderson's speech we could hear the admiration and respect for Michael and his family. Michael was so blessed to have such a wonderful doctor who cared so much.

Barry Borthistle compared Michael to Winston Churchill, saying that Michael is so strong and so focused in his message that it was possible to feel the positive energy in the air.

In Domenic's emotional speech, as he was holding back the tears, he said, "I wouldn't want any of you to imagine or go through what our family has gone through in the past few years. But we made it because of Michael." When Domenic said these words, Gloria burst into tears. It was therapeutic for her to release these pent-up feelings. Even though Michael was doing well, he was still in such a grey area as far as his health was concerned. The wounds from the ordeal Michael and the family had been through were still fresh.

Everyone in the room was experiencing mixed emotions— happiness that Michael had survived and accomplished so much, but sorrow for what he had been forced to endure. Love and support for Michael and our family filled the room. Many of the guests commented on the rush of emotion they had felt when Gloria broke down—there was intense realization among the crowd of just how devastating cancer had been for our family.

Michael was a tower of strength throughout the evening. His composure was amazing to see. This night was a dream come true for Michael. His goals were being realized. His CD was produced. His Foundation was being established, and he had been given the means to raise money for cancer research.

Between tickets, the auction, and a raffle, a total of $15,750 was raised for the Michael Cuccione Foundation. We decided to make this dinner an annual event, and we hoped that Alex would be able to attend many of them.

The celebration of Michael's CD Release Party was televised on BCTV, and Dr. Anderson and Michael were interviewed on CKNW.

One day, when Michael was at our family doctor's office, the doctor remarked to Michael that he was very lucky to be alive. "Five years ago there was no treatment for your type of relapse, but now, thanks to the research being carried on, people are surviving through the means that saved you."

Our hope is that in the next five years, if enough support is given to cancer research, others will survive because they, too, have been given the means.

Funds raised in Canada by the Michael Cuccione Foundation will be allocated to cancer research programs within Canada. A similar mandate to keep funds in the country in which they are raised will be applied throughout the world.

Chapter 16

Spreading The Message Across Canada

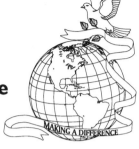

 Jan. 4, 1997

Domenic, Gloria, and Michael boarded a Norwegian cruise ship at San Juan, Puerto Rico for a one-week Caribbean cruise arranged for them by Barry Borthistle of Enrich International. It was Michael's 12th birthday today, and Domenic's is tomorrow. What a great way for them to celebrate their birthdays together!

 Jan. 5, 1997

This morning, Domenic, Gloria, and Michael were given a warm welcome by Enrich International members at their meeting in the Stardust Lounge, where Michael was guest speaker. The guests were from around the world. What a fantastic opportunity it was to spread his message. Barry Borthistle gave a powerful introduction of Michael. Everyone gave Michael a standing ovation as he approached the stage. Michael thanked Barry Borthistle for his incredible generosity in presenting him and his parents with this luxurious cruise.

Michael reflected on his illness and how the suffering of those around him had made him determined to help do something to put an end to it. He was grateful for the support of Enrich for his cause. Michael described the herbs he was taking and how much he felt they had helped him recover from his illness. Michael chose to sing *Make a Difference* because he felt that this was what everyone was trying to do. He received another standing ovation.

Michael's CDs were on sale. He raised over $1,200 through their sales, which he later deposited into the newly formed The Michael Cuccione Foundation.

During the cruise, Michael met Mark Victor Hansen, co-author of the best-selling *Chicken Soup For The Soul* series, a collection of inspirational stories written by the people who lived them. Mark Victor Hansen approached Michael and told him how impressed he was with Michael's story and his heartfelt way of delivering it. Hearing Mark Victor Hansen speak, Michael admired his powerful message and his inspirational stories.

Domenic, Gloria, and Michael had the time of their lives on this trip. The activities were endless, the ports of call were beautiful, and the food was unbelievable.

Michael asked Domenic to play bingo with him while Gloria was packing to go home. Michael picked out the cards. This was the last game of the evening, and the winners' pot held $1,600. Michael was thrilled beyond belief when Domenic's card was one of the two winners to split the pot. It was quite a send-off!

 Jan. 15, 1997

Michael and his parents have been busy since they arrived home. Michael was asked to visit several schools in the community to tell his story. He visited his elementary school today. He showed the video portraying the highs and lows of what he has experienced since he was diagnosed with cancer. He asked the audience: "How many of you have been touched by cancer in one way or another?" It was very shocking for Michael to see the number of hands that were raised.

Michael responded, "This is why I am helping to raise money for cancer research—so that no more hands will be raised in the future."

The school children were impressed with Michael's speaking ability and the courage he had shown throughout his ordeal.

 Jan. 18, 1997

Michael has made it to his 12th birthday! After all he has been through, Domenic and Gloria wanted to make this a very special birthday for him. They arranged for a bus to take Michael and his friends to Planet Hollywood for dinner.

The children had a terrific time together. The manager at Planet Hollywood recognized Michael and praised him for his many accomplishments. He presented Michael with a gift. When Michael opened up the gift bag, his mouth dropped in surprise. It was a classic Planet Hollywood jacket. What a special night!

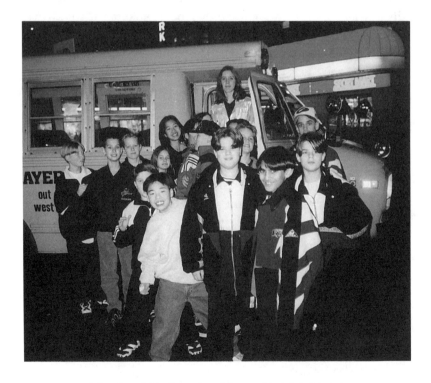

Michael and his friends celebrate his 12th birthday.

Feb. 5, 1997

Michael's recurrent sore throats have been causing us great concern, for Michael's succumbing to Hodgkin's disease had been preceded by severe bouts of strep throat. It's been decided to have his tonsils and adenoids removed with the hope of stopping his throat problems. Michael is thankful that the surgery will be performed soon, so that he can recover before the school's spring vacation.

 Feb. 18, 1997

Michael's tonsils and adenoids were removed. Obviously, they were in very bad shape. The surgeon had to remove a considerable amount of tissue and do extensive cauterization of the surgical site.

 Feb. 28, 1997

I am glad to see Michael eating properly. The surgery left him unable to eat much in the past ten days. He has lost over ten pounds.

 Mar. 10, 1997

Michael was eager to return to karate, after being inactive following the tonsillectomy. Unfortunately, when he was attempting to do a flying side-kick, he lost his balance and broke his right foot along the side of his little toe. I couldn't believe it when I went upstairs and saw him stretched out on the couch, crutches propped up against the wall. He has brought in a new meaning for "spring break."

Michael's broken foot hasn't slowed him down for long. Michael is lined up to appear on *Canada AM, The Dini Petty Show, Jane Hawtin Live,* and *100 Huntley Street* from April 7th to the 11th. Anna Terrana, East Vancouver MP and a dear friend of the Cuccione family, has made arrangements for

Michael to meet with the Right Honourable Prime Minister Jean Chrétien in Ottawa on April 10.

 Mar. 14, 1997

Gloria has been in contact with The Peoples Network (TPN) in Dallas, Texas, and has sent them a package containing Michael's video, newspaper clippings, and one of his CDs. TPN was so impressed that they ordered 600 CDs. They also requested that Michael attend their convention in Texas in June, 1997.

Michael's CDs were selling fast. Over 10,000 had been sold, and in excess of $65,000 had been raised for the Michael Cuccione Foundation.

 Mar. 23, 1997

Domenic, Gloria, and Michael met with the officials from Shoppers Drug Mart to see if Shoppers would sponsor the sales of Michael's CD across Canada. Michael gave the presentation, explaining his mission, and what it would mean to him to have their support. A video showing his experiences of the previous two years was shown.

After Michael's presentation, the people from Shoppers Drug Mart head office immediately made a commitment to help. They believed that Michael *will* make a difference. Michael is delighted that they have agreed to sell his CDs across Canada.

 Mar. 27, 1997

Domenic, Gloria, Michael, and Steven went to the Parliament Buildings in Victoria, B.C. to meet with the Premier of British Columbia. The ultimate purpose of this trip was to gain support for Michael's cause. They met with Premier Glen Clark and some of the staff, who were all very supportive. Media coverage of Michael and the Premier was broadcast on BCTV news and in the newspaper.

 Apr. 2, 1997

Enrich International have asked to have Michael speak at their convention in Orlando, Florida, in August. He is pleased to be asked to speak for a second time. The children will be out of school for the summer vacation, so Domenic and Gloria have made a decision to take the whole family.

 Apr. 5, 1997

Domenic, Gloria, and Michael flew to Toronto. Michael has started on his media campaign across Canada. Dini Petty made arrangements for them to stay at the Royal York Hotel in downtown Toronto. They'll spend the weekend visiting with relatives who live in the area.

 Apr. 7, 1997

Dini Petty sent a limousine to the hotel to take Domenic, Gloria, and Michael to the recording studios where *The Dini Petty Show* was being taped with a live audience. The show will air tomorrow.

Michael sang part of *Never Give Up*. Dini Petty said if anyone wanted to hear the rest of it, they could purchase the CD to help Michael raise funds for cancer research!

The first question Dini asked Michael was, "Did you ever feel like giving up?"

Michael replied, "There were times when I thought my life would be cut short, but I knew that my faith, my positive attitude, and the support from my family and friends would get me through just about anything."

Dini Petty then introduced another Hodgkin's survivor. He and Michael were interviewed together. The two of them shared their experiences regarding Hodgkin's disease, and talked about how setting goals had been a part of their recovery.

Michael was also interviewed on the radio for the *Jane Hawtin Live* show, and he appeared on an Italian TV program called *Telelatino*. Here he met the president of the Candlelighters, a support group for people recently diagnosed with cancer. She was highly impressed by Michael and invited him to join in their walkathon on August 20, 1997. He was also invited to be guest speaker at their convention in Montreal in the summer of 1998.

 Apr. 9, 1997

Michael appeared on *100 Huntley Street*. After a video showing his experiences of the past three years, he was interviewed. Michael must have impressed the interviewer, who suggested that in about 20 years he would be pleased to have Michael for a son-in-law!

Michael discussed the theological aspect of his experience with the interviewer. Michael has always given God credit for his survival and acknowledges Him in his speeches.

Michael closed the program by singing *Never Give Up*. The camera panned the audience, and showed Domenic and Gloria. I could see their love for Michael written on their faces as they watched him sing.

 Apr. 10, 1997

Today was the highlight of Michael's trip. At ten in the morning, Domenic, Gloria, and Michael flew to Ottawa to meet Prime Minister Jean Chrétien. A taxi took them to the House of Commons, where they were met by Anna Terrana. She introduced them to various officials as she showed them around the building. They had lunch in the same restaurant where the officials dined. They attended a session of the

legislature where tributes were paid to Michael by
Anna Terrana, and Sharon Hayes, MP for Port Moody-
Coquitlam.

Michael met with Prime Minister Jean Chrétien in his
office at three o'clock. Their rapport was immediate. The
Prime Minister had a great sense of humour. He chatted with
Michael for about 15 minutes. There was considerable media
coverage in the newspapers and on television of Prime

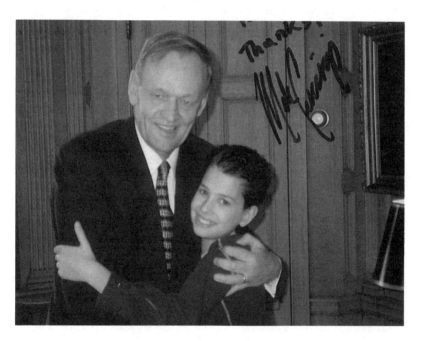

Michael gains support from the
Prime Minister of Canada.

Minister Jean Chrétien asking Michael if he (the Prime
Minister) was a was "a bad guy or a good guy."

Michael never missed a beat as he replied, "Obviously, you
are a very good guy." Then, Michael urged everyone to vote
for Prime Minister Jean Chrétien in the up-coming election.
With a big smile, the Prime Minister hugged Michael, and
jokingly requested that the 12 year-old be signed up to assist
with his election campaign!

When Michael expressed the need for federal government support of cancer research, the Prime Minister said that he was working on plans along these lines.

He was true to his word. At the end of June, 1997, Prime Minister Jean Chrétien announced on national television that his government would be funding 200 Canadian researchers across Canada, in the amount of $60 million, to work on finding a cancer vaccine. Michael is eternally grateful to the Prime Minister for his interest in, and support of, cancer research.

 Apr. 11, 1997

Michael was interviewed on *Canada AM*. Again, Michael told his story and sang *Never Give Up*. Calls came in from people praising Michael and wanting to hear more of his music. He was also interviewed on *Global News*. He was profiled on *Kid's Beat,* which was shown across Canada. Michael also received tremendous support from the Italian community. He was featured in several Italian papers every day that week.

The extensive media coverage is helping Michael to carry his message across Canada. Michael's mission to raise funds for cancer research is certainly working.

 Apr. 12, 1997

Domenic, Gloria, and Michael attended a family wedding in Toronto before returning home. Domenic and Gloria's wedding anniversary is today, so this was a great way to celebrate.

Apr. 13, 1997

Domenic, Gloria, and Michael returned home today with a lot to tell us. I am amazed at the amount of ground Michael has covered in the past two years since his bone marrow transplant.

 Apr. 19, 1997

Domenic and Gloria have gone on a trip to Las Vegas with other relatives. This is the first time that they have been away without the children since Michael became ill. I am taking care of the children while they are gone.

Today, Michael attended the 45th anniversary dinner for the researchers and pediatric doctors of Children's Hospital. Charlene Dryburgh, a member of the Board of Directors for the Michael Cuccione Foundation, offered to escort Michael to this event.

Following dinner, Michael addressed the group, and expressed his admiration to the doctors for their dedication to their work. He entertained everyone by singing two of his songs. The doctors involved in Michael's cancer treatments were utterly amazed that he was able to make this appearance, let alone that he looked so well.

Charlene told us later how much she had enjoyed the evening in Michael's presence. On the drive home, she had seen yet another side of him: that of Michael as a sibling. This aspect of him came out as Michael recited to her the speech he had recently written about Sophia, his teen-age sister. Charlene had been in stitches, especially when Michael reached the part of the speech where Sophia was using two portable phones—at the same time—one on each ear. Apparently, while in the washroom, Sophia had dropped one of the phones into the toilet. Of course, it wasn't her own phone. It had been the family phone!

It was no surprise to any of us, including Charlene, that Michael had won the School District Public Speaking Award for this speech.

Apr. 20, 1997

I took Michael and Steven to Kast Hair Studio. Michael's hairdresser, Mandy, had been so impressed by Michael's story that she arranged a cut-a-thon to raise funds for the Michael Cuccione Foundation.

Michael chatted and mingled with people as he autographed his CDs. He inspired adults and children alike to get involved in making this a successful event. Line dancers, face painters, and clowns provided entertainment throughout the day. Michael's little friend Ryan, a six year old, even got into the act. Dressed as a clown, he enjoyed his first-ever volunteer experience. He handed out balloons to everyone who stopped by to support Michael's cause. There was much laughter and fun for everyone involved.

Michael was interviewed live on an Italian radio station, and a picture of him getting his hair cut was featured in a local paper. Over $1,400 was raised at this event. The hairdressers at the salon plan to do this annually. It is terrific to see the local community supporting Michael.

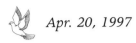 *Apr. 22, 1997*

Tonight Michael received *The Leaders of Tomorrow Award* presented by Volunteer Vancouver. This award honours people for their outstanding volunteer activity. It acknowledges that through the volunteering of their time they are contributing greatly to the benefit of the community. Michael, at age 12, was the youngest-ever recipient of this award!

It was so exciting to see Michael receiving such a prestigious award and being recognized for all his efforts! It was a perfect evening. On the way home, Michael wanted a snack, so we stopped at Domenic's parents for cold cuts. It's great to see Michael eating so well and gaining weight.

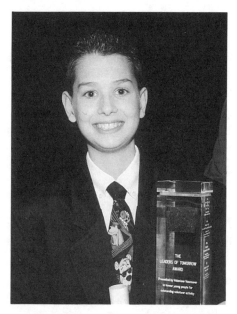

The youngest-ever recipient of the
Leader of Tomorrow Award.

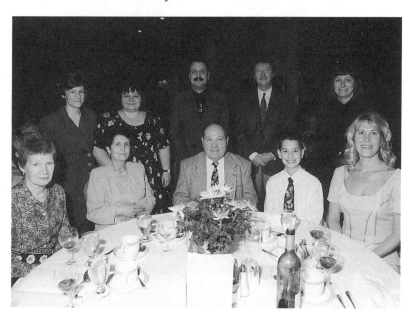

Michael surrounded by family and friends at The Leader of Tomorrow Awards Banquet.
(Front) L to R: Grandma Jane, Nonna Anna, Nonno Armando, Michael, Gloria
(Back) L to R: Charlene, Rose, Domenic, Greg, Sheryl

June 1, 1997

Michael appeared on the B.C.'s Children's Hospital telethon. He promised his signed CDs to the first 50 people who phoned in with a pledge of $50. His phone never stopped ringing! He had the honour of sitting on the celebrity panel between Sherry Ulrich, a singer, and Rick Hansen, another true hero.

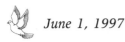 *June 3, 1997*

Gloria, Michael, Steven and I were invited to Planet Hollywood, where David Hasselhoff was making an appearance. He was in Vancouver to make a movie called *Nick Fury*. Planet Hollywood was sponsoring a contest. The winner would receive the opportunity to appear on the set of *Baywatch* for a day. Michael could certainly attest to the thrill of being able to do that!

After the contest winner had been congratulated by David, Michael went up to David and greeted him. David turned around and his eyes lit up as he saw Michael. He exclaimed to the cast members, "This is the boy I've been telling you about. He is the one who has raised over $65,000 for cancer research." Then he started singing *Never Give Up*! Michael was utterly amazed that David remembered these details of Michael's life.

When David and the cast in his movie went upstairs to be interviewed by the media, Gloria, Michael, and Steven were invited to join them. Lisa Rinna, David's co-star, asked Michael if she could have one of his autographed CDs. Naturally, he was only too happy to give her one. David requested another one, too. He said his five-year-old daughter was crazy about Michael's music and was always playing it.

David asked Michael if he remembered hearing about Charlie, the boy with terminal cancer who had spent so much time on the *Baywatch* set. He told Michael that Charlie had passed away in January. Charlie had made such a strong impression on everyone at *Baywatch*, David said they had been planning a *Baywatch* episode combining elements of Charlie's life story and Michael's song, *Make a Difference*. David offered Michael the starring role. . . he could be playing the role of Charlie! David said that Michael would have to do a screen test for the part of Charlie. They would be faxing Michael the dialogue from a couple of scenes for the test. David asked Michael if he had any experience in acting. Michael told him about the pilot parts he had acted in. David said he knew that it would be "a piece of cake" for Michael to fulfill the role.

Not wanting to take up any more of David's time, Michael wisely told his mother that it was time for them to go back downstairs. David continued signing autographs for boys and girls who had been waiting excitedly to see him.

Michael left for Dallas the next day a happy boy. There was the prospect of a *Baywatch* episode, plus another goal of gaining worldwide support was being realized. His message would be broadcast throughout the United States.

Chapter 17

Crossing Into The United States

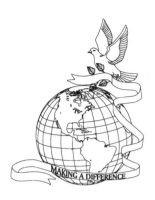

 June 4, 1997

This was a very busy day for Michael and Gloria. Michael's agent had called the night before for Michael to audition for a public service filming for *Youth Against Violence* at 9 a.m. Michael had a call-back for a commercial at 10 a.m., then they had to catch the plane to Dallas at noon. It is a good thing that Gloria can beat anyone for finding shortcuts in reaching destinations. They made all their appointments right on schedule.

In Dallas, a shuttle service whisked them to their hotel. At 7:30 p.m., Gloria phoned Domenic to let him know that they had arrived safely. Domenic had received Michael's lines for his *Baywatch* screen test. I forwarded them so Michael could practise while he was away.

 June 5, 1997

Gloria and Michael went to the opening ceremonies of the Dallas Convention for The Peoples Network (TPN) and were directed to the VIP area. They were overwhelmed when they entered the conference room—over 7,000 people were in attendance! A huge movie screen was on each side of a large stage. A fantastic sound system was playing the national anthem. After the national anthem was played, Gloria turned to Michael and asked him if he was nervous. Michael replied that he wasn't. He was taking everything in stride, which is characteristic of Michael. He was enjoying every minute of it and looking forward to making his appearance the next day.

In the meantime, Michael and his mother went sight seeing and shopping for gifts for the family. That evening, they dined at Planet Hollywood in Dallas.

 June 6, 1997

Mark Victor Hansen was one of the guest speakers today. Gloria and Michael were invited to meet backstage with him after he had finished speaking. Mark Victor Hansen remembered meeting Michael on the Caribbean cruise. Michael said that it looked like they were following one another from place to place. TPN had previously covered Michael's story on their motivational satellite-TV program. This was shown throughout the United States and Canada. Another one of Michael's dreams has come true.

It was Michael's turn to speak. Jeff and Eric, who were introducing the speakers, were talking about Michael as if he weren't expected. His video was shown, then Jeff came out and announced that they had a surprise guest. "Michael is here in person!"

When Michael strode onto the stage with his big smile and his eyes beaming, he received a standing ovation from the 7,000 participants. When the audience sat down, Michael said humbly, " Is this for me?"

Everyone laughed. Michael said that it was an honour for him to be there and that it was hard for him to watch the video, but he felt that his life had been spared for a reason. He had survived because of his faith and positive attitude, in conjunction with all the great medical care. He went on to say that it was through the support of organizations like TPN that he was able to make a difference. He described his illness and its effects on him and his loved ones, and emphasized that now was time for people to do something about the disease before it strikes one of their relatives or friends. He complimented TPN on their readiness to support worthy causes such as the fight against cancer. After a second standing ovation, Michael left the stage. Just before the next speaker was about to be introduced, Michael returned to the stage to present Jeff and Eric, founders of TPN, with a plaque which said: "It's people like you who make a difference in the world."

Jeff replied by saying that Michael was the first boy he had met who he would allow to date his daughter. The audience howled and Michael received another standing ovation.

Renee, Jeff's wife, helped set up Michael's CDs. Within three hours, over 600 CDs were sold. While Michael was autographing them, people told him about their experiences with cancer and how seeing Michael had changed their lives forever. A woman who had lost her ten-year-old son to cancer asked if she could give Michael a hug. Another woman had battled cancer, been in a tragic car accident resulting in a coma, survived a 20-foot fall, and was carrying on with life. She told Michael that he was an inspiration to *her!* This lady is a motivational speaker and is certainly making a difference by giving people the courage to never give up, despite their adversities.

After the meeting, Gloria and Michael raced to the Dallas airport to catch their flight home. They had to cut their trip short in order for Michael to fulfill a commitment to a cancer fundraiser called "Relay For A Friend". He was to participate in the candlelight closing ceremony by speaking and singing. On the way home, he and his mother practised the lines from the scenes for his upcoming screen test. They certainly had a full schedule.

 June 8, 1997

We received a call to tell us that Alex was dying. Alex has been so close to our family that it was natural for us to be together at this time if only to comfort his family. Domenic and Gloria were against Michael going to the hospital because they were afraid that it would be too traumatic for him. Michael insisted on going. I agreed with Michael because I believed that not experiencing this final time with Alex would have a worse effect on him. He would always feel that he had let Alex and his family down. But, when Gloria phoned back to ask if Alex could still hear what was being said to him, she was informed that he had just passed away.

They went straight to the hospital to be with the family. Michael bore up very well, stroking Alex and praying over him. Michael's calm demeanor when he arrived home told me that I had been right about him. Michael's presence had been a great comfort to Alex's mother. They had hugged one another warmly. She said to Michael, "I am going to make it. I'm not going to give up." They cried together.

Alex's nurse told Michael, "Hard as it is to believe, Alex enjoyed his last days. He was so inspired by you that he spoke of you all the time. I hope that you will keep fighting for this cause."

Michael replied that he was going to fight even harder. Steven was touched that Alex had even remembered his promise to give Steven the Canadian National Soccer jersey. Alex was this kind of man—always considerate of others.

One day, we may know why God allowed Alex to leave us so early in his life, but it is very difficult for us to accept now. He had so much to offer the world. He was going to university to be a lawyer, but after he'd developed leukemia and went into remission the first time, he began studying to be a doctor. He would have been a great one.

 June 12, 1997

Domenic, Gloria, and Michael had to go to the hospital today. Michael was having tests to determine if he is cancer-free after two years. So soon after Alex's death, we were even more apprehensive about the results. Michael had his blood work done and his chest x-ray taken. Later they met with Dr. Anderson to get the results of these tests.

Dr. Anderson knew it was important for us to have the results quickly because he understood how hard it was for us to have to wait. Dr. Anderson was smiling as he delivered the good news. Everything was great. Michael was cancer-free! He had passed another milestone.

Dr. Anderson did have something else to talk about, which was difficult. He was planning to move in order to begin practising at Children's Hospital in Calgary, Alberta. He had been offered a great position and was needed in Alberta. Dr. Anderson assured Michael that he would still be there for him. Michael was speechless. He will be receiving only one more check-up from Dr. Anderson.

Michael was pretty quiet as he went to have his pulmonary function test. When this was done, Michael and his parents met with the pulmonary specialist. Michael's pulmonary count was still only 51, when it should be 100. There has been no increase since the last test; on the other hand, there hasn't been a decrease. The specialist has kept Michael on pulmacourt, a steroid inhaler to help combat the inflammation and mucous in his lungs. He is still optimistic that Michael's lungs will become stronger in time. We can only pray that they do.

On the way home Michael showed how upset he is over the news of Dr. Anderson's leaving. He feels that he is not only losing a great doctor but also a good friend.

Later that night, Gloria and Michael prayed together. Michael came to the conclusion that Dr. Anderson must be really needed in Calgary, and that there is a reason for everything.

Dr. Anderson provided exceptional care for Michael ever since he was first diagnosed with Hodgkin's disease. He made calls to many parts of the world to find a protocol of drugs that would be most effective for Michael's disease. He was devastated when Michael's cancer returned. He knew that in order to save Michael's life, Michael would have to go through the chemotherapy, bone marrow transplant, and radiation treatments. His tears flowed freely when he informed Michael

and his parents about the treatments Michael would have to undergo. Dr. Anderson, more than anyone, knew about the risks involved, and the pain and suffering Michael would have to endure. We were extremely lucky to have such a skilled oncologist looking after Michael. His devoted care and compassion played a big part in helping to save Michael's life.

 June 16, 1997

Michael was given a main part in the television commercial called *Youth Against Violence*. He spent today shooting it. One of Michael's most admired Vancouver Canucks hockey players—Trevor Linden, who does so much charity work—was in the commercial with him. Michael was thrilled. Strange to say, even though Michael spent the last hour of the film supposedly running to escape some bullies, he arrived home full of energy. You would never know that he only had a pulmonary count of 51!

 June 17, 1997

Michael did the screen test for the part of "Charlie." It will be about a week before he will find out if the directors in Los Angeles approve of him for the part. Michael will also need clearance by the United States government to work in Los Angeles.

 June 24, 1997

We are all ecstatic for Michael. He definitely has the part of "Charlie" and he has been cleared to work in the United States. Filming will start about mid-July. It was made clear that the whole family was welcome. This is a thrill of a life time for the whole family!

Chapter 18

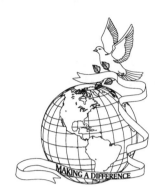

Michael Plays Charlie

Born in Santa Ana, California, Charlie Dodson Hays was diagnosed with medullary thyroid cancer in September 1991. He was given six months to live. After having an operation and radiation treatments, Charlie managed to live six years after his diagnosis. Charlie, with his younger brother Perry and their mother, Susan Addington, visited the California beach of Malibu before Charlie learned that his cancer had spread to his lungs and bones, about two years before his death. Charlie wanted to spend his last few months in Malibu. They were living in Park City, Utah, at the time. The tumours in his lungs were leaving him only 35 percent breathing capacity, but Charlie was able to breathe more easily near the ocean.

"This is heaven, this is where I want to live, and this is where I want to die, too," Charlie told his mother. She knew that she could not afford to stay in Malibu so she made a plan. She placed an advertisement in the Malibu Times, *offering to do housekeeping or look after children in return for accommodations for Charlie, Perry, and herself. A benefactor who wished to remain anonymous offered Susan and her sons a beach house for as long as it was needed. One of Charlie's last wishes had been granted.*

Interviews on 20/20 and Inside Edition *reveal how bravely and unselfishly Charlie dealt with crises in his life. These programs show how Charlie, on his 12th and last birthday, used his savings and the donations that he had received to purchase presents for sick children in the hospital. As ill as he was, he even delivered the gifts himself.*

As well, Charlie had allowed researchers to conduct tests on him. These tests resulted in the discovery of the mutant gene that led to Charlie's type of thyroid cancer. Because he had no doubt been responsible for saving lives through his courageous sacrifice, Charlie was given a lifeguard's memorial service after he died.

Charlie's mother and Gloria found the similarities between Charlie and Michael striking. When Susan watched videos of Charlie, Gloria and Michael were amazed. Charlie and Michael looked so much alike in pictures of their early childhood. Both were singing, dancing, and hamming it up, with big smiles on their faces. Their mothers, Susan and Gloria, resemble each other in appearance. Both boys had spent time on Baywatch, *where they had been welcomed royally. They had both known intense suffering, emotionally and physically. They each had a close friend who had been extremely loyal. Charlie used his experience with cancer to help humanity. Michael is trying to help fund a cure for cancer through his Foundation. Charlie was very spiritual and so is Michael.*

Michael would find it easy to play the part of Charlie. Michael felt that he knew Charlie already.

 July 9, 1997

Domenic, Gloria, Sophia, Michael, Steven, and the children's cousin, Armando, boarded a flight to Los Angeles, California. A shuttle bus met them at the airport and took them to their hotel.

They stayed in two adjoining rooms with a pool below their windows. When they entered their room, they spotted a basket of chocolates and other goodies addressed to Michael. A card from David Hasselhoff said, "You are going to have a ball and make a difference." Michael was delighted. It was a wonderful welcome!

After dinner, they received a call from Sheldon, a coordinator of events for David Hasselhoff, wanting to know if everything was satisfactory at the hotel. Lines from the episode "Charlie" were delivered to the room. Michael studied the whole script. He absorbed it thoroughly and was soon able to tell everyone in detail what it was about.

 July 10, 1997

In the afternoon, Domenic, Gloria, and Michael were taken to the *Baywatch* office by a crew member. Greg Bonann, executive producer and director, met with them. This was very exciting. Greg allowed Michael to look through one of the cameras while he was finishing off some filming. They were working in a tank of water to do some of their scenes.

Anita, David's publicist, came over and suggested that they go for lunch. After they ate, Anita gave Domenic, Gloria, and Michael a tour of the *Baywatch* office. That is when they met some of the *Baywatch* staff.

Michael went for some wardrobe fittings, then was taken to David's office to meet with him. It was great for Michael to see David again. David gave Domenic, Gloria, and Michael a warm reception, then discussed the script and some story line changes with Michael.

 July 11, 1997

Today was the big day. Michael started work. He was taken to his own trailer, which was furnished with all the conveniences of home. His wardrobe was laid out for him. Greg Bonann, the director, soon realized that Michael could handle the script. Michael felt confident with his lines, and responded to directions quickly, thus requiring few retakes.

 July 12 & 13, 1997

Michael had the weekend off to enjoy some sightseeing with his family. The family rented a car, toured the area, and visited Rodeo Drive. They did a little shopping and had lunch in one of the prestigious restaurants. The next day they went to Venice Beach, where numerous activities take place constantly. There were six blocks of interesting shops and restaurants. They were able to pick up some nice gifts and souvenirs along the way.

Sunday night, after going out for dinner, they returned to the hotel, where the children spent some time swimming in the pool. They went to bed fairly early, so Michael would be rested for the next day.

 July 14 – 21, 1997

During the week, the family was welcomed to spend time on the beach where they were filming the episode. They had a lot of fun with the cast. Michael was in most of the scenes and was really enjoying himself.

On Tuesday, David's publicist introduced the family to Susan Addington, Charlie's mother. They hugged each other and wept. The mothers instantly bonded through the mutual suffering they had experienced with their sons' illnesses.

Susan was happy that Michael was playing the part of Charlie. Michael resembled Charlie strongly in nature. He was so warm and loving, just as Charlie had been. When Susan embraced Michael, I am sure that for a few moments it was like she was holding Charlie again.

In the evening, the family was able to watch the dailies of Michael's performances. David Hasselhoff and Greg Bonann were very pleased with them. There was one funny incident which David is sending to *Bloopers*. Michael is holding a grunion fish tenderly in his hands. He looks at it solemnly before releasing it into the ocean with the words, "It's time for you to go home." Just as the fish is swimming away, a seagull swoops down and takes off with the fish in its mouth. Needless to say, that part was left out of the episode.

Wednesday was a day off for Michael. The family spent the day shopping for a plaque to give to David Hasselhoff and Greg Bonann, to show their appreciation for all they had done for Michael and the rest of the family. The plaque has these words:

> To David, Greg and the *Baywatch* family. Thank
> you for making a difference in my life and for
> making a worldwide awareness with Episode 8005
> (Charlie). One person can only do so much, but
> together we can make a difference.

Michael presented this plaque to David and Greg after he
had finished filming his part of the episode. They were very
moved by Michael's presentation.

David and Greg played the game Paper, Scissors, Rock to
see who got the plaque for the first year. David came out the
winner.

One day everyone joined in the celebration of David's
birthday. His wife, his two daughters, and his mother and
father came to the set. They brought a cake and everyone sang
"Happy Birthday" to David. It was an honour for Michael to
meet them.

Without question, playing the scene when Charlie dies was
hardest on Michael. He had faced death several times himself

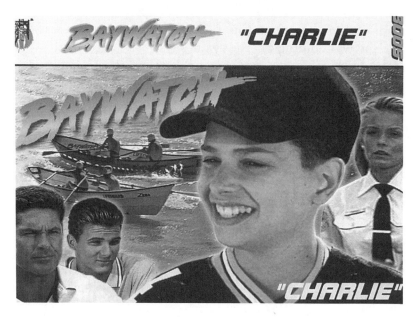

Michael portrays Charlie.

and had lost dear friends to cancer, but Michael reasoned that since the scene was only going to take a few minutes, he could control his emotions. He knew that Charlie would want this episode to inspire others. Michael was doing this scene for Charlie, Melinda, Stephanie, Alex, and everyone else suffering and dying. He, like Charlie, was going to do everything he could to prevent future suffering.

The final scene in the episode was Charlie's lifeguard memorial service. Lifeguards dressed in their uniforms were standing on the shore. Charlie's stage "mother" and "sister" were standing there with David Hasselhoff. The "sister" broke down where she paid tribute to Charlie, so David took over. He spoke of how Charlie had wanted to make a difference and had succeeded. He spoke of how Charlie was a true lifeguard because he was saving lives. He had allowed doctors to use his body and as a result they had isolated the gene that caused Charlie's type of thyroid cancer. David said that everyone was glad that Charlie had been with them. Then he choked as he mentioned Charlie's "wonderful smile." A beautiful wreath with Charlie's name on it was rowed to a waiting motor-boat. Reverently the wreath was placed on the water, where it floated into the distance. There was no re-take on this scene.

Susan had tears in her eyes through this part of the episode—as would any mother who had lost a beloved child.

A helicopter came down and did a curtsey in the water, splashing everyone around it. Susan said that Charlie was playing a joke on them, for this is something that Charlie would have thought was a big joke. When a rainbow unexpectedly appeared, Susan thought it was a sign of Charlie's approval of what was happening.

Charlie had been afraid that he would be forgotten. Susan is seeing that this does not happen. She has started Faces of Courage, The Charlie Hays Foundation.

The episode was completed sooner than expected so the family had another weekend of sightseeing. They went to Newport Beach for the day and to a restaurant for dinner. Hobie, the cast member who plays David's son, met with them to say good-bye.

On Tuesday morning, just before they left, a member of the staff from *Baywatch* delivered navy blue *Baywatch* jackets with their names on them. What a thoughtful thing to do! David phoned to say good-bye to everyone and commented on how happy he was with Michael's performance.

During the filming, David and Michael had appeared together for interviews on *Entertainment Tonight* and *Canada AM*, discussing the *Baywatch* episode about Charlie. There was some indication that the episode was a departure from the usual *Baywatch* episodes. David pointed out that they do several inspirational episodes a year. David himself gets involved in worthwhile causes internationally. Lives have been saved through people learning cardio-pulmonary resuscitation (CPR) by seeing it done on *Baywatch*. Valerie Pringle of *Canada AM* asked Michael if he could act. Michael replied, "Maybe you should ask David that question." David assured her that Michael could act. He wished that more actors were as eloquent as Michael.

 July 23, 1997

I have never seen Michael as happy as he was when he returned home after doing the "Charlie" episode on Baywatch. *He was pleased that he was able to accomplish the job. Michael was privileged to play the part of Charlie. I know that they would have been great friends. Michael was proud, too, that he and Charlie had been given the opportunity to make a difference, as* Baywatch *is viewed worldwide by millions of people.*

Michael had almost a month to enjoy the summer holidays with his friends before leaving for Florida. This was the first time in three years that Michael had been able to spend his summer doing things that boys his age enjoy. He went on sleep-overs, rode on all the rides at the Pacific National Exhibition playground, attended football games, went swimming and picnicking. In short, he did everything he had been wanting to do for so long. He and his family thoroughly enjoyed a five-day visit to Vancouver Island, to visit my son Phillip and his family. They went to Tent Island on Phillip's boat, where they had great fun beachcombing, hiking, and fishing. They went water-skiing on Shawnigan Lake and enjoyed the ferry rides to Vancouver Island and back. It was wonderful to see Michael smiling and looking so healthy. The Michael I knew so well was back!

Chapter 19

Continuing Michael's Mission

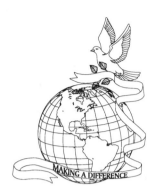

 Aug. 20 – 28, 1997

Michael and his parents have left for Orlando, Florida, where Michael will speak at the Enrich International Convention. They had been so impressed by Michael's presentation on the Caribbean cruise that they wanted him to speak a second time. Michael cannot believe that he will be sharing the stage with such celebrities as Barbara Bush!

When Michael walked out on the stage, he received a standing ovation from over 3,000 people. He updated everyone on the progress that had occurred in less than a year in his health, much of which he felt was due to Enrich herbs. He told how he had gone from 59 pounds to 100 pounds in the past two years, and had more energy than ever.

He also informed the audience about what he was doing to spread his message. He cited one of his creeds: "If we all try to make a difference, each day, imagine the big difference that will be made in a very short time." He talked about the Foundation and how it had been able to raise over $140,000 in one year.

He told the audience about how he had been honoured to portray Charlie in an episode of *Baywatch*. He was thankful to David Hasselhoff for giving him this opportunity, for it continued the message he and Charlie have for the world.

He mentioned that he had been touring local schools, showing the video of his story and his experiences with cancer. He said that he was amazed at how many children had been touched by cancer in one way or another. "This is why we have to join together in the fight against this disease," Michael emphasized.

He went on to say that he had told the children that having cancer does not necessarily mean a death sentence. People are recovering due to the research that has been done in finding a cure for cancer. He expressed his hope that, through fundraising, more researchers can be funded so that one day this disease will be a thing of the past. He closed by singing one of his songs. His CDs sold out so he took orders for more.

At the convention, Enrich International offered an interesting sales competition for their distributors. For reaching $1 million in total sales that weekend, the corporation held a draw for a Mercedes Benz. The winner shrieked with joy when she heard her name announced. And if $1.5 million in total sales were reached, Barry Borthistle had agreed to have his head shaved, symbolic of Michael's earlier hair loss. They reached this objective, too—an indication of how valued by the public these herbs are. He had to be shorn, and as he was, Barry remarked, "You are enjoying this, aren't you, Michael?"

That night, the family attended a dinner provided by Enrich International. Beginning the next day, the family spent the rest of the time visiting Disney World. They enjoyed the rides and amusement activities, went to water parks with wave pools, water slides, and sandy beaches.

 Aug. 28, 1997

The family returned from their incredible trip.

 Sept. 2, 1997

The children have returned to school. Steven is in Grade 4, Michael is in Grade 7, and Sophia in Grade 10.

Michael loves his new school. He is attending what is known as a middle school. This school has classes for

Grades 6, 7 and 8. He has a great homeroom teacher and he is really looking forward to participating in sports. He has been chosen to be vice-president of the school. There is certainly a difference in how school is going for Michael this year!

 Sept. 17 – 19, 1997

Accompanied by his father and mother, Michael left school for several days to continue his cancer research promotions. Michael seems to have little difficulty catching up with his school work when he returns from these trips. His teachers are very understanding about providing him with work that he can do while travelling.

The first stop was Calgary, Alberta, where they stayed for two days. Domenic, Gloria, and Michael were delighted to see Dr. Anderson again.

Michael's first appearance was scheduled at the Science Centre in Calgary, where he met with the Bank of Montreal Employees Society. Dr. Anderson was invited to introduce Michael.

The Society showed their video of the various charities they support, one of which is The Michael Cuccione Foundation. Their video showed excerpts of Michael's story as well.

He performed one of his songs and Dr. Anderson commented to Michael on how his voice had matured and how well he was singing.

Michael was amazed when this society presented him with a $5,000 cheque payable to the Michael Cuccione Foundation. This was a potent indicator of their belief in Michael's cause, for the Bank of Montreal Employees Society is highly selective in causes that they choose to support.

Domenic, Gloria, and Michael went to visit Gloria's friend Lori, in the Foothills Hospital, where she was receiving more chemotherapy in preparation for the harvesting of her stem cells. Ahead of her was the bone marrow transplant itself. She appreciated the assistance she received from Dr. Anderson in regard to her medical treatment.

Michael and his parents also visited Children's Hospital in Calgary, where Dr. Anderson is now practising. Dr. Anderson gave them a tour of the hospital and introduced them to the staff researchers. There was a baby there who had been born with a cancerous tumour on its foot. The parents were terribly upset. Gloria and Michael tried to offer some comfort and Michael gave the parents one of his CDs.

Later, Domenic, Gloria, and Michael were invited to visit Dr. Anderson and his family at their new home. They had a wonderful visit.

Michael was also busy doing interviews. He appeared on two TV stations and one radio station, and there was a write-up about him in the local newspaper.

Michael and his parents flew to Toronto yesterday. Today Michael went on a walkathon, a fundraiser for Candlelighters, the support group for newly diagnosed children with cancer, and their families. The walkathon ended up at City Hall, where Michael spoke, then sang *Never Give Up*.

 Sept. 21, 1997

The family went to St. Peter's Church today, where Michael spoke to everyone present about how his faith helped him beat cancer. "The Lord is just a prayer away," he stated. I am sure that he was an inspiration to all, including the priests, who were obvious in their admiration. Again his CDs were completely sold out.

 Sept. 22, 1997

Today is Gloria's birthday and Michael appeared on *Doctors On Call,* which airs on TV stations across Canada. They discussed cancer in general and Hodgkin's disease in particular. The callers to the show were very taken by Michael's story. A friend from British Columbia called in to the show to say how much the words in Michael's songs have helped her family because her daughter is battling leukemia.

Michael also did an interview with *CHIN,* which is an Italian TV station. He spoke of his determination to help find a cure for cancer. The TV show host presented Michael with a T-shirt and Michael gave him one of his CDs. An account of this interview and other stories involving Michael appeared in the *Toronto Star* newspaper.

 Sept. 23, 1997

Michael and two of his cousins saw the Stanley Cup at the Hockey Hall of Fame. They had lunch there and played the video games.

Michael was also interviewed again on *Telatino,* the Italian TV program. The Italian papers updated Michael's progress since the last time he was in Toronto.

 Sept. 25, 1997

Gloria and Michael flew to Orlando, Florida, while Domenic flew home to be with Sophia and Steven.

Michael has been invited to speak at the Netcorp Travel Convention. Netcorp is a multi-level marketing travel agency. They heard about Michael through TPN. They chose the Michael Cuccione Foundation as the first non-profit organization for which they hoped to raise funds. The president of the company introduced Michael to some other children. Michael enjoyed the time spent with them.

Gloria and Michael toured Universal Studios and went on all the rides. In the evening they attended the Netcorp welcoming dinner. All the guests were treated to a trip to Pleasure Island where they spent the evening having a fun time.

 Sept. 27, 1997

Michael did a presentation for Netcorp. The audience was deeply touched with his heartwarming story. He was given a $1,000 donation for the Foundation. In the evening, Gloria and Michael attended a farewell dinner. Later on, Michael got together with friends for pizza.

Before returning home, Michael and his mother visited MGM Studios. Michael convinced Gloria to join him in the elevator-type ride called the Tower of Terror. Michael went in it three times. Gloria declined to go again. Once was enough!

 Sept. 29, 1997

Michael returned to school and settled back into his usual routine. He believes in his mission and is prepared to dedicate his life to it, but I am sure that he appreciates it when he can spend some time doing things that boys his age enjoy.

 Oct. 9, 1997

This was a day we were still feeling a bit of anxiety about. Michael had his usual three-month tests. He received a clean bill of health except for his pulmonary count, which is still 51. There has been no increase since the last tests. The specialist feels that it could be two years before there is any significant increase. We all hope that the radiation treatments have not damaged his lungs permanently. He is two inches taller and has gained six pounds, which brings him up to 100 pounds. Michael's blood test were great. His hemoglobin was 149, his white blood cell count was 9.61, his red blood cell count was 5.31, and his blood platelets are 285. He can now start going for his tests every six months, instead of every three months. This is truly a relief.

 Oct. 17 – 19, 1997

The Cuccione family was invited to the premiere of the episode "Charlie". It was held in Los Angeles and attended by Gloria, Sophia and her friend Tracy, Michael, and his friend Brodie. On October 17, the day of the event, they attended a barbecue. There were over 200 people in attendance. Michael met Chad, Charlie's devoted friend, who was still very upset over Charlie's death. Charlie's mother felt that getting Chad and Michael together with Michael would be healing for Chad.

Later, Chad, Brodie, and Michael enjoyed time together. Sophia and Tracy were having an exciting night talking to the *Baywatch* cast and getting autographs. Michael's music was playing in the background. There was a table of items for sale such as Michael's CDs and tapes, "Charlie" videos and T-shirts.

The guest speakers that evening were David Hasselhoff, Tai Collins, scriptwriter; Greg Bonann, executive director; and Charlie's mother, Susan Addington. David surprised Michael with a lifeguard's rescue cannon autographed by all the *Baywatch* cast. On top of the cannon was an envelope containing a $10,000 cheque donated to the Michael Cuccione Foundation by David and Pamela Hasselhoff. Michael and his family were ecstatic!

Michael was unusually nervous when the "Charlie" episode was shown. He wanted so much to have done a good job of portraying Charlie. Everyone, including the producers, felt that Michael had done a great job.

 Nov. 8, 1997

When "Charlie" was aired in November, it was enthusiastically received. Many people who watched it told us how moved they were by the story and Michael's portrayal of "Charlie." Michael was such a natural. The episode featured Michael's song, *Make a Difference*, and ended with a dedication to both Charlie and Michael.

Following the airing of the Baywatch *episode, Michael received numerous letters of support for his cause and requests for his CDs.*

As soon as Gloria and Michael returned, they started preparing for the next big event: the Second Annual Fundraiser for the Michael Cuccione Foundation. This would be held at the Italian Cultural Centre on November 21. Michael wrote two new songs to sing at the event: Whether Life Is Sun Or Rain *and* Learning From The Best. *He feels that in the past three years he has learned much from everyone.*

Chapter 20

The Second Annual Michael Cuccione Foundation Fundraiser

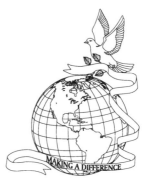

Domenic and Gloria and the Board of Directors put a lot of effort into making the Second Annual Michael Cuccione Foundation Fundraiser a success. They could have sold over a thousand tickets if the facility could have accommodated the people. All the guests eagerly anticipated the evening. It was wonderful to see how the support for Michael and the Foundation had grown.

 Nov. 21, 1997

Tonight was the big night. It was a formal affair and everyone looked fabulous. Michael was handsome in his tuxedo. The doors opened at 6 p.m. and the excitement began. As the guests came through the doors, many embraced Michael and his family with hugs of support. Everyone seemed ready to celebrate.

There were tables laden with silent auction items, which were donated by numerous supportive companies. People crowded around the tables, placing their bids excitedly and checking from time to time to see that they were not out-bid.

Before the guests entered the main hall they were each greeted and presented with a box of chocolates donated by Hershey's Chocolates. This company is assisting in the launch of a school fundraiser for the Michael Cuccione Foundation.

The hall looked wonderful, lit up by lights streaming from floor to ceiling. The stage was surrounded with greenery and more lights. Tables of guests filled the room.

A program outlining the events of the evening was placed at each table setting. The Cuccione family portrait on the cover of the program symbolized how working together as a family had helped them make it through trying times. The newly designed Foundation logo represents Michael's intent to carry his message worldwide, with Michael's own words in bold letters: **"One person can only do so much, but together we can make a difference."**

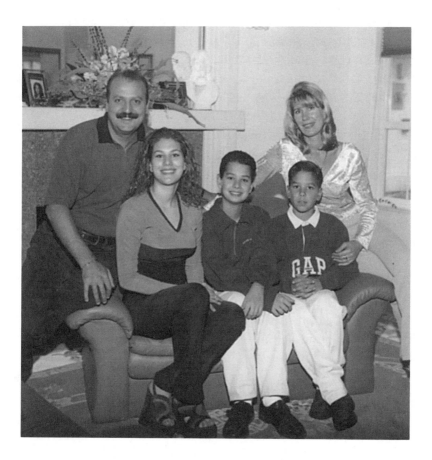

The Cuccione Family in 1997
L to R: Domenic, Sophia (15 yrs), Michael (12 yrs), Steven (9 yrs), Gloria.

So much happened during the evening. Michael dedicated the celebration to the seven special people who are no longer with us. *In Loving Memory* was shown, a video of these seven people, the events in Michael's life before and after his cancer, and Michael's accomplishments through the last year. The song *No Tears In Heaven* by Eric Clapton could be heard in the background. The life and death struggle with cancer was made very real in this video. It is clear why Michael is working so hard to make a difference.

After the video and opening, dinner was served and the formal program began. Marke Driesschen of Global TV was master of ceremonies. He has a great sense of humour and was obvious in his admiration of Michael. He was amazed that a boy of twelve years old could have accomplished so much in such a short time. He and Michael made a great team.

Dana Cole, Michael's voice teacher, sang and dedicated to Michael the song *One Moment in Time*. She called Michael up to the stage so she could have him by her side. This song carries a lot of meaning for Michael, and it was even more special to have Dana sing it to him. Michael had come into Dana's life around the same time she lost her mother to cancer. They are very close. It seems that, in one way or another, we have all been touched by cancer.

Michael Cuccione, Sr., president of the Foundation and Michael's uncle, was one of the guest speakers. He thanked everyone for showing their support through their attendance. He assured those present that the Foundation would keep them informed as to where their donations were going and of the latest developments in the research work being financed by the Foundation. He asked God to bless everyone with good health.

Major sponsors' representatives were guest speakers. They were Sheryl O'Toole, Category Coordinator for Shoppers Drug Mart, and Mike Lacombe from Burger King. (Mike is also vice-president of the Michael Cuccione Foundation.)

Dr. A. Tingle, Director of BC Research on Child and Family Health, was a special guest speaker. He enlightened everyone about what was being done in the way of research for childhood cancer.

It was Michael's turn to speak. He was introduced by Marke. Everyone simultaneously stood on their feet and applauded Michael as he made his way up to the stage. We could feel a tremendous amount of love and admiration in the room. What a difference a year makes! Michael looked so well. He started his talk by thanking God for his health: "He was always there for me when I needed Someone to talk to." He went on to thank his parents, family, friends, and sponsors for their support. Michael told about his unbelievable year, mentioning his travels to Los Angeles, Orlando, Dallas, Toronto, and Calgary, and the excitement of doing the "Charlie" episode on *Baywatch*. He said how special it was to have met the Prime Minister of Canada.

Michael also spoke very highly of David Hasselhoff and the *Baywatch* family. They are people Michael will never forget. David and his wife, Pamela, were so generous in their gift of $10,000 to the Michael Cuccione Foundation. Michael was also grateful for having the numerous opportunities to spread his message at all the conventions and national radio and television talk shows throughout the year.

There were many out-of-town guests in attendance who had come in especially for this night. Michael was particularly pleased that Alex's father, Peter, and Alex's sister from Alberta were able to attend. Alex's mother was still too grief-stricken over the loss of her son to come with them. Alex's father explained how hard it was for them to attend, but he knew Alex would want him to be there for Michael. Gloria felt that towards the end of the evening a great sense of peace came over Alex's dad. Although he shed many tears, it seemed to comfort him to be part of Michael's special evening because he knew that Michael and Alex had admired each other so much.

During the evening there was a live auction, followed by raffle and door prize draws. Michael joined in, helping by displaying the items. Domenic's aunt and uncle won the trip for two to any destination of their choice in North America. We were all happy for them.

Michael made three presentations that evening. The first was a glass clock for Marke Driesschen, thanking him for the fine job he had done as master of ceremonies. Dr. Anderson was very surprised when he was also called up and presented with a glass clock with an inscription saying: "You are the best doctor in the world to me. Love, Michael." Michael went on to say that Dr. Anderson had played a big part in his being here tonight: "I believe that times like these make Dr. Anderson's job worthwhile." Dr. Anderson was touched by Michael's obvious respect and affection for him.

Then Michael called up Dr. Tingle and the staff from B.C.'s Children's Hospital. He asked Dr. Anderson to return to the stage. Michael astounded the audience by announcing that the Michael Cuccione Foundation was donating $50,000 to

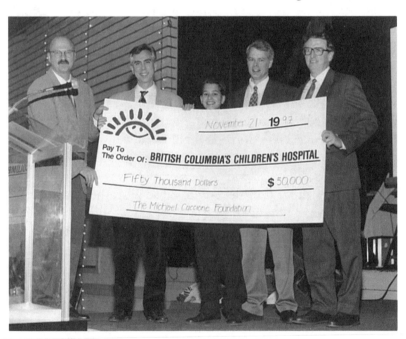

Michael presenting the $50,000 cheque.
L to R: Marke Driesschen, Dr. Schultz, Michael Cuccione,
Dr. Anderson, Dr. Tingle

B.C.'s Children's Hospital Foundation. This was the first installment toward establishing the Michael Cuccione Foundation Fellowship. The aim is to continue to contribute to a $500,000 endowment fund to hire a full-time cancer researcher and support hospital programs dedicated to cancer research.

As Michael handed the $50,000 cheque to Dr. Tingle, he was extremely proud. This was concrete evidence that he was moving toward his target. What an incredible accomplishment for a twelve-year-old boy!

We later received a letter from the president of B.C.'s Children's Hospital Foundation extending deepest appreciation to Michael and the Michael Cuccione Foundation. She further stated that this donation will be "a lasting legacy in Michael's name" and would help the more than 1,000 cancer patients seen each year at this hospital alone.

Anna Terrana, former MP for Vancouver East, came up to make a special announcement. The Right Honourable Jean Chrétien, Prime Minister of Canada, had sent a letter to show his support for Michael. This meant so much to Michael because with the government's support and funding we can reach our goals a lot faster. The letter reads:

It gives me great pleasure to extend my greetings to everyone gathered here for the Second Annual Michael Cuccione Foundation Fundraiser. While advances have been made in the early detection and treatment of cancer, there is still a great deal to be done. The ongoing promotion and support of research are vital to continuing this progress. The Michael Cuccione Foundation—in their fundraising and information

*initiatives—certainly recognizes this, and so too does
the Government of Canada. On June 25th, I was proud
to announce a partnership between our government and
Pasteur Merieux Connaught Canada. Under Technology
Partnerships Canada, we are investing $60 million in a
project to find a cancer vaccine—representing the
largest biotechnology investment ever made in Canada.
This will allow Pasteur Merieux Connaught Canada to
assume a world mandate to develop, produce, and
export worldwide, therapeutic vaccines to combat the
seven forms of cancer that account for 66 percent of all
cases in Canada.*

*With every step taken, we get closer to beating
cancer. It is very much a collective effort and the
Michael Cuccione Foundation can be commended for its
contributions. I would be terribly remiss if I did not
acknowledge the person behind today's event. In
Michael Cuccione, we have an individual whose
unstinting efforts in support of cancer research have
helped to promote awareness of a disease he has faced
so bravely over the course of his young life. His
exemplary courage and determination deserve our
admiration and respect.*

*Please accept my kindest regards,
Jean Chrétien
Prime Minister of Canada*

We were amazed that the Prime Minister would take the
time to write such a warm and friendly letter in time for
Michael's special evening. It was reassuring to all of us to
know that our Prime Minister is so interested in trying to find
a cure for cancer. He paid such a glowing tribute to Michael.
We know that he was most sincere in his praise.

Michael ended his presentation by performing one of his
two new songs, called *Learning From The Best*. While Michael
was travelling and making contact with many people, he felt

that they were learning from each other. He expressed his feelings in these words: *You inspire me, I inspire you.*

While Michael was announcing the winners of the silent auction, a guest took it upon himself to collect money from the other guests sitting at his table to donate to Michael's cause. He then challenged other tables to match or better the donations. This started a chain reaction with other tables of guests joining. A great deal of money was raised this way.

Michael sang his second new song, *Whether Life Is Sun Or Rain*. In this song he is comparing life to weather: *Life and weather never stays the same.*

The band started playing and the dancing began. Michael visited with his guests and danced with his family and friends for the rest of the evening.

Incredibly, over $32,000 for the Michael Cuccione Foundation was raised at the Second Annual Fundraiser. This amount more than doubled the funds raised at the first event. The warmth and love for Michael and the support for his cause was simply outstanding!

 Nov. 26, 1997

We received another exciting letter from Ottawa today. It follows:

> *On behalf of the Right Honorable Jean Chrétien, I wish to thank you for your recent letter. I trust that your fundraiser was a success, and that the message from the Prime Minister was received in good order. In discussing the event with your mother, I indicated that I would see to it that further information on the government's involvement in cancer research would be forwarded to your attention. To that end, I have sent copies of your correspondence to the Honourable John Manley, Minister of Industry, and the Honourable Allan Rock, Minister of Health. I am sure they will appreciate being made aware of your efforts and will respond to you directly.*

The Prime Minister has asked that I extend his kindest regards to you and your family.

Sincerely,
Mark Stokes
Manager, Correspondence

Michael was delighted with the support offered in the letters sent from Jean Chrétien and Mark Stokes. Imagine someone as busy as our Prime Minister taking the time to acknowledge Michael's endeavours!

 Jan. 5, 1998

Yesterday was Domenic's 43rd birthday and today is Michael's 13th birthday. All the family gathered together to celebrate. Each time Michael celebrates another birthday it is especially meaningful to all of us.

Another reason to celebrate is that our friend Lori is in total remission! We are overjoyed to hear this uplifting news. Another survivor!

After the family had gone to bed, Michael went into Domenic and Gloria's bedroom.

"Could we have a birthday prayer?" he asked.

"Sure, would you like to start it?" Gloria replied.

"No, you go ahead." Michael said.

Gloria started the prayer. Halfway through, Michael added, "Thank you, God, for helping me to make it to my 13th birthday. When I was ten years old I wondered if I would make it to my next birthday. I pray that you will help me to make it to my 43rd birthday, like my dad."

What does the future hold for Michael? It is hard to say. Only God knows the answer to that one. One thing for certain, Michael will continue to keep campaigning for cancer research. As Michael says, "I am not stopping here. I am keeping on until a cure for cancer is found." We all pray that God will give him the strength to do this.

Chapter 21

Michael's Songs and Their Meanings To Him

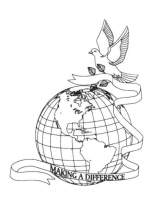

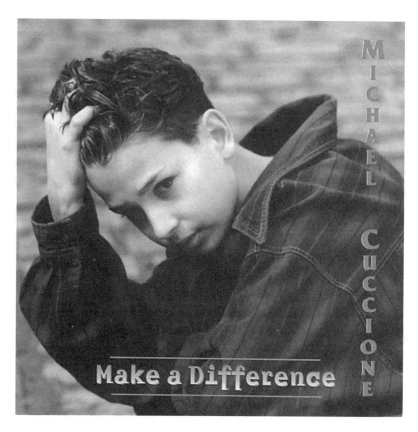

Cover of Michael's CD.

WHEN YOU ARE AWAY

When you are away
When you cannot stay
I miss you when you are gone
When I hear you through the night
I know everything is going to be all right
When I wake up and see your sight
It's almost like seeing the light

When you are away
I wish that you were here
I miss those happy cheers
When you are away
Why couldn't you be near
Day and night it feels so right

You know that I love you
And I know that you love me too
I know all that we've been through
And that prayer can come true

I know it hasn't been fair
But you always show you care
I feel things are turning around
Soon we'll be back on solid ground

This song was written for my dad's 40th birthday. It tells about how much I missed him when he was at work and couldn't be with me in the hospital. I have also lost friends to cancer and really miss them now they are gone.

MAKE A DIFFERENCE

I wanna make a difference in this world
Reach out to the sky
See a difference in my eye
To make the difference in this world
May God make the tears drift away

Make a difference in this world
Tell the boys and the girls

I wanna make a difference in this world
If we all do our part we can make a brand new start
To make a difference in this world
Let's try to understand and reach a hand
I wanna make a difference in this world
I want to stay strong and see things come along

To make a difference in this world
I feel in my soul we can't go wrong
Make a difference in this world
I feel in my soul, we can't go wrong.

This one is expressing what I want to do and how I believe this will happen.

I DON'T WANNA SAY GOOD-BYE

I don't wanna say good-bye
I don't wanna make you cry
Why do people come and go
When there is so much love to show
I don't wanna say good-bye
I don't wanna make you cry

Because our love can be so true
There is so much I wanna do
You know how much I care
Love in life is to share
Day by day, year by year

I am going to stay right here
Forever is not a choice
One day we will hear God's voice
And I hope today is not the day
Because right now I wanna stay
I don't wanna say goodbye
I don't wanna make you cry

This was written when my cancer came back for the second time and I faced the possibility that I might have to say good-bye. I knew what this would do to those who love me and how this would interfere with my plans for the future. I had so much that I wanted to accomplish.

LOCK THE DOOR

When I wake up in the morning
The morning light
I feel something minor
A minor fright
I've been through this feeling a few times before
And now I know what to do
I am going to lock the door

When the going is rough
When times are tough
I am going to lock the door
Not having any more
I know what we've gone through now we're fine
Show happiness and love all the time
Life means more today then ever before

And now I know what to do I am going to lock the door
Life can be cruel but also kind
What I've seen people go through blows my mind
If you think about the good your day will shine
And that's why I am gonna take one day at a time

    I wrote this song after my second bout with cancer. This song gave me the strength to believe that I had locked the door on my disease for good.

NEVER GIVE UP

Dreams they are for dreaming
Life you know is for living
It takes a lot of caring
To make your dreams come true
Many things are bound to happen
To you and to me
Stop blaming all the reasons
Why this could be
Never give up on hope
Never give up on faith
Never give up on love

When suffering does not seem
To have an end
Positivity is the answer
Fight till the end
When you are feeling scared and lonely
And need someone there
Just know in your heart

There are people who care
Never give up on hope
Never give up on faith
Never give up on love

I know sometimes life
Doesn't seem too promising
Be strong in your heart and in your mind
Even in your hardest times you could imagine

Don't you ever

You just never give up on life
Never give up on hope
Never give up on faith
Never give up on love

This song is what I believe in. This is my philosophy in life: *You have to care if your dreams are going to come true.* Even if bad things happen, you have to keep on going and not blame anything or anyone. Remain positive and know that there are people who care. Dreams are for dreaming and life is for living. I have worked hard to make my dreams come true. I never gave up on hope, I never gave up on faith, and I never gave up on love.

Chapter 22

Michael's Goals

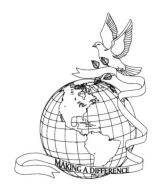

Michael knows and understands all of the challenges associated with cancer treatments. His own experiences, and his inspiring leadership and dedication, have given him the motivation and true desire to help other people beat cancer.

Michael has made the commitment to help stop the pain and suffering. With his own unique talents and brave heart, he has dedicated his life to creating an awareness for the need to find a cure. He wants to encourage people to stay positive, to never give up, and to never stop working for this important cause.

He wants to carry this message worldwide.

Chapter 23

About the Foundation

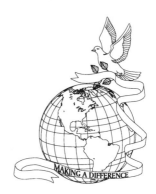

The Michael Cuccione Foundation was incorporated under the Society Act of British Columbia, on March 12, 1997 and achieved charitable status on June 18, 1997.

The purposes of the Foundation are as follows:

- To raise funds, receive bequests, gifts and voluntary donations of every kind and accumulate a fund, and to expend or administer this fund or the proceeds thereof, or the income from the fund, exclusively for cancer research and for the use of children's hospitals located in Canada.
- To raise the awareness of the need to fund cancer research.
- In order to inspire others to assist with the Foundation's cause, to conduct motivational speaking engagements at schools, at businesses, and at different levels of government.
- To provide emotional support to cancer patients and their families.
- To organize an annual dinner/dance, an annual golf tournament, and other events including bake sales, bottle drives, hair cut-a-thons, and car washes.
- To promote all these activities throughout Canada and the world.
- Michael and the Board of Directors will monitor the use of the funds. This information will be made public through Michael's website: **www.makingadifference.org**.

By the end of 1997, the Michael Cuccione Foundation had raised over $170,000 for cancer research.

Part of the proceeds from the sales of this book will be donated to the Michael Cuccione Foundation.

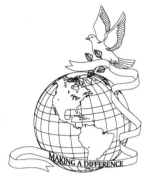

For Further Information

The Michael Cuccione Foundation
P.O. Box 31081
8 - 2929 St. Johns Street
Port Moody, British Columbia
Canada   V3H 4T4

Phone/Fax: (604) 552-2850
E-mail: love@makingadifference.org
E-mail: support@makingadifference.org
http://www.makingadifference.org

To order copies of this book, *There Are Survivors: The Michael Cuccione Story,* or Michael's *Make a Difference* CD or tape, please use the order form on the next page.

To mail a donation to Michael's cause, please make your cheque or money order payable to *The Michael Cuccione Foundation* and forward it to:

The Michael Cuccione Foundation
P.O. Box 31081
8 - 2929 St. Johns Street
Port Moody, British Columbia
Canada   V3H 4T4

To make a donation using VISA or MasterCard, please complete the form on the next page and forward it to The Michael Cuccione Foundation.

Donations can also be made through Michael's website: **http//www.makingadifference.org**

Income tax receipts will be issued for donations over $20. For donations under $20, receipts will be provided upon request.

Thank you for helping Michael to
Make A Difference!

ORDER FORM

Item Description	Qty.	Price	Subtotal
There Are Survivors: The Michael Cuccione Story (Soft cover book)		$19.95 (Cdn)	
Make a Difference - Compact Disc		$12.00 (Cdn)	
Make a Difference - Cassette Tape		$10.00 (Cdn)	
		Merchandise Total	
		Shipping & Handling	
		SUBTOTAL	
		GST: Add 7% of Subtotal	
		(No PST on books) **PST**: Add 7 % (BC) of Subtotal 8 % (Ont) 6.5% of GST Subtotal (Que)	
		GRAND TOTAL Add GST Subtotal (and PST if Applicable)	

Shipping & Handling

Add the Shipping Charge below to the merchandise total (Canadian Rates)

Merchandise Item	**Shipping***
Soft cover Book	$5.00 for first book Add $3.00 for each additional book
CD or Cassette Tape	$2.00 for first CD or Tape Add $1.00 for each additional CD/Tape

---

Please send me these selected products. Enclosed is: Cheque ☐ Money Order ☐ Please charge my: Visa ☐ MasterCard ☐
Please make cheques payable to *Making A Difference Publishing*.
Card # _____ Expiry _____ Signature _____

Name (please print) _____ Company Name _____
Address _____
City _____ Province _____
Postal Code _____ Home Phone_____ Business Phone_____
Shipping Address if different from above
_____

Mail order form with payment to: *Making A Difference Publishing*
P. O. Box 31081, 8 - 2929 St. Johns Street
Port Moody, BC Canada V3H 4T4
Phone/Fax: (604) 552-2850

YES! I want to help Michael make a difference!
Please find enclosed my contribution of: ☐ $100 ☐ $75 ☐ $50 ☐ $25 ☐ Other $ _____
Enclosed is: Cheque ☐ Money Order ☐ Please charge my: Visa ☐ MasterCard ☐
Please make cheques payable to *The Michael Cuccione Foundation*.
Card # _____ Expiry _____ Signature _____

Name (please print) _____ Company Name _____
Address _____
City _____ Province _____
Postal Code _____ Home Phone_____ Business Phone _____

Mail donation and form to: *The Michael Cuccione Foundation*
P. O. Box 31081, 8 - 2929 St. Johns Street
Port Moody, British Columbia
Canada V3H 4T4

Thank you for your order and support!